D1784578

ROBERT A. SMITH, DVM, MS
CONSULTING EDITOR

THE VETERINARY CLINICS

OF NORTH AMERICA

FOOD ANIMAL PRACTICE

Biosecurity of Cattle Operations

DAVID A. DARGATZ, DVM, PhD, GUEST EDITOR

VOLUME 18 • NUMBER 1 • MARCH 2002

W.B. SAUNDERS COMPANY
A Division of Elsevier Science
PHILADELPHIA   LONDON   TORONTO   MONTREAL   SYDNEY   TOKYO

W.B. SAUNDERS COMPANY
A Division of Elsevier Science

The Curtis Center • Independence Square West • Philadelphia, Pennsylvania 19106

http://www.wbsaunders.com

THE VETERINARY CLINICS OF NORTH AMERICA: Volume 18, Number 1
FOOD ANIMAL PRACTICE   ISSN 0749-0720
March 2002
Editor: John Vassallo

The Veterinary Clinics of North America: Food Animal Practice (ISSN 0749-0720) is published bimonthly by W.B. Saunders Company. Corporate and editorial offices: The Curtis Center, Independence Square West, Philadelphia, PA 19106-3399. Accounting and circulation offices: 6277 Sea Harbor Drive, Orlando, FL 32887-4800. Periodicals postage paid at Orlando, FL 32862, and additional mailing offices. Subscription prices are $104.00 per year for US individuals, $143.00 per year for US institutions, $52.00 per year for US students and residents, $124.00 per year for Canadian individuals, $187.00 per year for Canadian insti-tutions, $141.00 per year for international individuals, $187.00 per year for international institutions and $71.00 per year for Canadian and foreign students/residents. To receive student/resident rate, orders must be accompanied by name of affiliated institution, date of term, and the *signature* of program/residency coordinator on institution letterhead. Orders will be billed at individual rate until proof of status is received. Foreign air speed delivery is included in all *Clinics* subscription prices. All prices are subject to change without notice. POSTMASTER: Send address changes to *The Veterinary Clinics of North America: Food Animal Practice*, W.B. Saunders Company, Periodicals Fulfillment, Orlando, FL 32887-4800. **Customer Service: 1-800-654-2452 (US). From outside of the US, call 1-407-345-4000. E-mail: hhspcs@harcourt.com**

The Veterinary Clinics of North America: Food Animal Practice is covered in *Current Contents/Agriculture, Biology and Environmental Sciences, Index Medicus,* and *Excerpta Medica.*

Printed in the United States of America.

CONSULTING EDITOR

ROBERT A. SMITH, DVM, MS, Diplomate, American Board of Veterinary Practitioners; and Associate Professor and McCasland Foundation Chair, Department of Veterinary Clinical Sciences, Oklahoma State University College of Veterinary Medicine, Stillwater, Oklahoma

GUEST EDITOR

David A. Dargatz, DVM, PhD, Diplomate, American College of Theriogenology; Epidemiologist, United States Department of Agriculture, Animal and Plant Health Inspection Service, Veterinary Services, Centers for Epidemiology and Animal Health, Fort Collins, Colorado

CONTRIBUTORS

GEORGE M. BARRINGTON, DVM, PhD, Diplomate, American College of Veterinary Internal Medicine; Assistant Professor, Department of Veterinary Clinical Sciences, College of Veterinary Medicine, Washington State University, Pullman, Washington

ROBERT J. CALLAN, DVM, PhD, Diplomate, American College of Veterinary Medicine, Assistant Professor, Integrated Livestock Management Program, Department of Clinical Sciences, College of Veterinary Medicine and Biomedical Sciences, Colorado State University, Fort Collins, Colorado

DAVID A. DARGATZ, DVM, PhD, Diplomate, American College of Theriogenology; Epidemiologist, United States Department of Agriculture, Animal and Plant Health Inspection Service, Veterinary Services, Centers for Epidemiology and Animal Health, Fort Collins, Colorado

SCOTT DEE, DVM, PhD, Diplomate, American College of Veterinary Microbiologists; Department of Clinical and Population Sciences, University of Minnesota, College of Veterinary Medicine, St. Paul, Minnesota

R. PAGE DINSMORE, DVM, Diplomate, American Board of Veterinary Practitioners; Associate Professor, Department of Clinical Sciences, College of Veterinary Medicine and Biomedical Sciences, Colorado State University, Fort Collins, Colorado

JAMES F. EVERMANN, MS, PhD, Professor, Department of Veterinary Clinical Sciences, College of Veterinary Medicine, Washington State University, Pullman, Washington

FRANKLYN B. GARRY, DVM, MS, Diplomate, American College of Veterinary Internal Medicine; Professor and Coordinator, Integrated Livestock Management Program, Department of Clinical Sciences, College of Veterinary Medicine and Biomedical Sciences, Colorado State University, Fort Collins, Colorado

JOHN M. GAY, DVM, PhD, Diplomate, American College of Veterinary Preventive Medicine; Associate Professor, Department of Veterinary Clinical Sciences, College of Veterinary Medicine, Washington State University, Pullman, Washington

DAVID P. GNAD, DVM, Assistant Professor, Veterinary Medical Teaching Hospital, Kansas State University, Manhattan, Kansas

SANDRA GODDEN, BSC, DVM, DVsc, Department of Clinical and Population Sciences, University of Minnesota, College of Veterinary Medicine, St. Paul, Minnesota

WILLIAM D. HUESTON, DVM, PhD, Diplomate, American College of Veterinary Preventive Medicine (Epidemiology); Professor of Epidemiology, Center for Animal Health and Food Safety, College of Veterinary Medicine, University of Minnesota, St. Paul, Minnesota

BRIAN J. McCLUSKEY, DVM, MS, Diplomate, American College of Veterinary Preventive Medicine; Epidemiologist, United States Department of Agriculture, Animal and Plant Health Inspection Service, Veterinary Services, Centers for Epidemiology and Animal Health, Fort Collins, Colorado

PAUL S. MORLEY, DVM, PhD, Diplomate, American College of Veterinary Internal Medicine; Director of Biosecurity, Veterinary Teaching Hospital, Colorado State University, Fort Collins, Colorado

MICHAEL W. SANDERSON, DVM, MS, Diplomate, American College of Theriogenology; Associate Professor, Department of Clinical Sciences, Kansas State University, Manhattan, Kansas

DAVID R. SMITH, DVM, PhD, Diplomate, American College of Veterinary Preventive Medicine (Epidemiology); Diplomate, American Board of Veterinary Practitioners, Food Animal Practice; Assistant Professor, Department of Veterinary and Biomedical Sciences, Institute of Agriculture and Natural Resources, University of Nebraska–Lincoln, Lincoln, Nebraska

JARED D. TAYLOR, DVM candidate 2002, Virginia-Maryland Regional College of Veterinary Medicine, Blacksburg, Virginia

JOSIE L. TRAUB-DARGATZ, DVM, MS, Diplomate, American College of Veterinary Internal Medicine; Professor of Equine Medicine, Department of Clinical Sciences, College of Veterinary Medicine and Biomedical Sciences, Colorado State University, Fort Collins, Colorado

SCOTT J. WELLS, DVM, PhD, Diplomate, American College of Veterinary Preventive Medicine; Department of Clinical and Population Sciences, University of Minnesota, College of Veterinary Medicine, St. Paul, Minnesota

CONTENTS

in cattle populations, it is informative to review principles of biosecurity from another livestock species in which these issues have been considered (e.g., swine) and compare these perspectives to the current situation for cattle. The authors follow a biosecurity risk-assessment model to identify important health hazards, evaluate risks, and present principles for implementing a cattle biosecurity program for important gastrointestinal health hazards of adult dairy cattle, after consideration of a swine biosecurity model.

There are many forms of respiratory disease in cattle. The most common is Bovine Respiratory Disease Complex, which is a multifactorial infectious disease that ultimately manifests as bacterial bronchopneumonia. Prevention of this common and costly disease problem requires an integrated management approach that improves animal resistance to infection and decreases animal exposure to pathogens. Biosecurity management is one aspect of respiratory disease prevention, but there are several biosecurity principles that have been historically underutilized. Improving biosecurity management of BRD should help reduce the prevalence and cost of this problem. This paper will focus on bovine respiratory disease although the principles discussed are equally applicable to other food animal species.

Application of rational principles of risk management in designing an effective biosecurity plan for reproductive diseases can be an important part of a profitable operation. Knowledge of the disease status of the particular herd, the effective strategies for disease exclusion including test performance and reservoirs is necessary. Development and implementation of a biosecurity program is an individualized effort undertaken for a particular operation. Knowledge of the disease status of the herd for each agent of concern and prioritization of the diseases most important in the herd is necessary. The biosecurity plan is then specific for the herd and the particular agent(s) of concern. Practitioners can apply knowledge of the epidemiology and ecology of disease agents to identify and implement logical control points for the individual herd.

Arthropod-borne diseases (ABD) of cattle include those pathogens transmitted mechanically and biologically from one bovine to another or from other species to cattle. This article provides examples of the more common ABD of North America and reviews strategies to prevent entry of ABD onto cattle operations and control transmission of ABD once established on cattle operations using an integrated approach.

Biosecurity for Mammary Diseases in Dairy Cattle 115
R. Page Dinsmore

Today's dairy farms are expanding at an unprecedented rate. Introducing new cattle to an existing herd during expansion increases greatly the risk that contagious mastitis pathogens such as *Streptococcus agalactiae*, *Staphylococcus aureus*, or *Mycoplasma* spp will be introduced as well. However, the most recent USDA/NAHMS survey (Dairy '96) indicated that fewer than 5% of herds quarantine introduced cattle, and fewer than 10% culture milk samples from introduced cows before commingling them. In this article, the above three contagious mastitis pathogens are described, with particular attention paid to the methods of introduction and spread of these infections. Various screening procedures are discussed, and protocols are suggested to minimize the risk that expanding herds will experience outbreaks of contagious mastitis.

Biosecurity of Veterinary Practices 133
Paul S. Morley

Hospitalization of sick animals tremendously increases their risk of acquiring infections as this congregates animals that are most likely to be shedding infectious agents with animals that often have enhanced susceptibility. In order to provide the best veterinary care possible, veterinarians have an underlying responsibility to minimize the risk of additional harm that might unintentionally befall a patient because of their interventions. This includes minimizing the risk of exposing patients to infectious agents. It is therefore incumbent upon veterinarians to actively manage the risk of nosocomial infections. Nosocomial infections in veterinary hospitals are not solely a patient-care concern; the spread of infectious agents can also significantly impact normal hospital operations, revenue, client confidence, public image, and can even affect the morale of hospital personnel. In some cases nosocomial agents can also be zoonotic. This paper discusses the need for biosecurity programs in veterinary practices, and describes a practical approach for developing biosecurity practices that are tailored to individual facilities.

Epidemiological Tools for Biosecurity and Biocontainment 157
David R. Smith

Sometimes biosecurity or biocontainment strategies that seem like a good idea end up being ineffective or inefficient in actual practice. Quantitative models are useful for predicting outcomes. Epidemiological principles and probability theory have been used to model the expected outcomes of biosecurity or biocontainment actions. This article shows how veterinarians can use computer spreadsheet software to test-drive biosecurity plans under a variety of "what if?" scenarios before the actions are implemented.

The bovine practitioner has a critical role to play in promoting biosecurity at both the farm level and the national level. Successful exclusion of exotic diseases, biocontainment of endemic diseases, and emergency preparedness rest soundly on bovine practitioners as part of the national biosecurity team. Bovine practitioners must voice their opinions on the strengths and weaknesses of existing and proposed national biosecurity programs. Healthy debate about national biosecurity programs and consideration of biosecurity issues by national veterinary organizations provide valuable feedback for the continual improvement of the programs and enhance their credibility. The health and productivity of US agriculture depend on national biosecurity.

FORTHCOMING ISSUES

RECENT ISSUES

VISIT OUR WEB SITE

For more information about Clinics:
http://www.wbsaunders.com

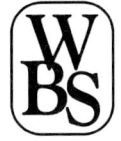

THE VETERINARY
CLINICS
Food Animal
Practice

Vet Clin Food Anim 18 (2002) xi–xii

Preface

Biosecurity of cattle operations

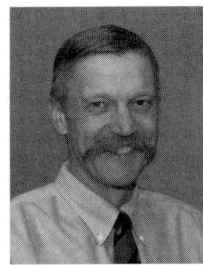

David A. Dargatz, DVM, PhD
Guest Editor

Over the past three to five years biosecurity has become a more commonly used word, first with veterinary professionals and then more recently with the media that serve the agriculture community. This increased awareness and focus of attention was initially the result of the livestock industries working to deal with diseases for which there are no vaccines or the vaccines have serious limitations. In addition, as herd sizes continue to grow, often through the acquisition of new animals from off-farm sources, producers and their veterinarians become keenly aware of the risks of introduction of disease agents onto the operation. More recently, outbreaks of diseases not currently present in the United States have caused everyone to think about how such diseases might be introduced into the country. Finally, speculation about the potential of intentional introduction of disease agents has raised awareness and concern even higher.

The authors of the chapters in this issue of the Veterinary Clinics of North America: Food Animal Practice hope it will provide the veterinary practitioner with a framework for developing and customizing biosecurity programs directed at controlling certain types of infectious disease agents. The practitioner will not find a detailed prescription for programs for every operation in their practice because the physical facilities, function and operation of each facility varies extensively, and thus the biosecurity and biocontainment programs must be tailored to each specific situation. The information in the following chapters will provide a framework for developing biosecurity and biocontainment programs for cattle operations and veterinary clinics.

I am indebted to the authors of the chapters in this issue for making the effort to share their extensive expertise in the field of infectious disease control for cattle operations. I also greatly appreciate the patience and expertise of the W. B. Saunders staff in helping to bring the issue together.

David A. Dargatz, DVM, PhD
United States Department of Agriculture
Animal and Plant Health Inspection Service
Veterinary Services
Centers for Epidemiology and Animal Health
555 South Howes Street
Fort Collins, CO 80521, USA

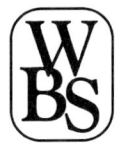

THE VETERINARY
CLINICS
Food Animal
Practice

Vet Clin Food Anim 18 (2002) 1–5

An introduction to biosecurity of cattle operations

David A. Dargatz, DVM, PhD[a],*,
Franklyn B. Garry, DVM, MS[b],
Josie L. Traub-Dargatz, DVM, MS[b]

[a]US Department of Agriculture, Animal and Plant Health Inspection Service,
Veterinary Services, Centers for Epidemiology and Animal Health,
555 South Howes Street, Fort Collins, CO 80521, USA
[b]Department of Clinical Sciences, College of Veterinary Medicine
and Biomedical Sciences, Colorado State University,
300 West Drake Road, Fort Collins, CO 80523, USA

The emphasis of this introductory article is to familiarize the reader with the terminology and broad concepts of biosecurity and biocontainment. This issue of the *Veterinary Clinics of North America: Food Animal Practice* has been prepared to provide a framework of considerations in developing biosecurity plans focused on various types of disease agents that may be introduced into or spread within cattle operations.

Definition of biosecurity and biocontainment

Biosecurity is the outcome of all activities undertaken by an entity to preclude the introduction of disease agents into an area that one is trying to protect [3,7]. For example, entities involved in developing biosecurity plans range from the national government to an individual farm operator and include all the levels in between. Disease agents of interest may include infectious agents and noninfectious agents such as toxicants. The area being protected by a biosecurity plan might be the nation, a region, or a local farm operation. The control of disease agents that are already present on a farm operation (e.g., precluding the transfer to new groups of animals) is usually called *biocontainment*.

---

* Corresponding author.
E-mail address: David.A.Dargatz@aphis.usda.gov (D.A. Dargatz).

Historical perspective and background on biosecurity

Interest in and discussion of biosecurity have expanded immensely in recent years. Much of this heightened awareness has been driven by world events, such as the occurrence of bovine spongiform encephalopathy in the United Kingdom and outbreaks of foot-and-mouth disease around the world. Other trends that have stimulated more interest in biosecurity are the changing demographics of agricultural operations, the disease agents being considered for control, and other concerns about the use of disease control technologies in livestock operations. Cattle operations in the United States continue to grow larger. In many cases, especially for dairy operations, the rate of expansion of individual operations is beyond what can be supported by internal replacement, so operations have been forced to introduce animals or, in some cases, whole herds from outside sources into their existing production system. Furthermore, cattle operations have become more specialized, focusing on the production of beef or milk and purchasing more of their inputs, such as feeds, from other specialized operations. The reliance on external inputs to the system leads to a loss of direct control of the production of those inputs and the potential that those inputs contain disease agents such as *Salmonella*.

Some of the disease agents of interest, including respiratory pathogens, require a multifaceted approach to control. Some infectious disease agents, including certain clostridial diseases, have been controllable using a single strategy such as vaccination. There are no effective vaccines, however, to protect against disease agents such as *Mycobacterium avium* subsp. *paratuberculosis*. This also applies to many of the food safety pathogens, including *Salmonella* spp. and *Escherichia coli*. To deal with disease agents in the harvest and postharvest arena, the Hazard Analysis and Critical Control Point (HACCP) approach has been adopted.

There is also concern regarding the use of chemical agents for the control of diseases and production in livestock populations. Antimicrobial resistance is a growing issue in human clinical medicine [1,4,5]. The role that antimicrobial use in animals plays in the emergence of resistant human pathogens is unknown; however, livestock producers and veterinarians are being encouraged to use antimicrobials judiciously to preserve the effectiveness of antimicrobials in veterinary and human health care settings [2]. Part of the judicious-use principles call for an emphasis on disease prevention. Disease prevention activities take into account the epidemiologic triad for disease occurrence. The triad consists of the individual host or animal, the disease agent, and the environment. One must recognize that the activities that affect the arms of the triad are potentially synergistic. Activities directed at improving specific or nonspecific immunity of the host may improve the ability of the host to resist the introduction of the agent if exposure occurs. Activities directed at the agent are primarily meant to limit the exposure of the host to the agent. Activities directed at environmental management also limit the potential risk that the agent will be sustained in the environment at an adequate level to result in animal disease. All of these activities are potential components of a biosecurity plan.

Most of the well-defined biosecurity programs in which livestock producers and veterinarians have become involved up to the present time have been those organized or mandated by government agencies. Examples include the tuberculosis, brucellosis, hog cholera, and pseudorabies eradication programs. For these programs, there was a broadly based conviction that the producers' livelihoods and the public were best served by organizing, funding, and enforcing strict disease control guidelines through government intervention. Similarly, considerable effort and resources are applied toward maintaining national freedom from numerous foreign animal diseases that currently are not present in the United States. For the numerous reasons just cited, it seems that circumstances are developing that make voluntary, producer-specific biosecurity programs increasingly attractive. Such individualized programs could be beneficial to the producer. One clear benefit of well-designed health management programs that incorporate biosecurity and biocontainment principles is the reduction of costly disease problems and enhancement of productivity and profitability. Beyond that, food safety concerns and the development of trace-back systems and accountability systems may provide additional compelling reasons for producers to document that risk reduction steps have been implemented, similar to the HACCP programs used by food processors. These efforts may be particularly important for producers seeking new markets for their livestock and other products. A challenge for the future will be analyses of cost-benefit and risk-benefit ratios for specific disease or pathogen reduction programs.

The concepts of biosecurity are not new. Without question, technologic advances in the areas of vaccinology, therapeutic drugs, and diagnostic testing have improved our ability to control disease immensely. Even before these recent advances, however, there were remarkable efforts and successes in the control of some diseases. In 1892, contagious bovine pleuropneumonia was eradicated from the United States [6]. This eradication occurred 6 years before the etiologic agent was identified as a *Mycoplasma* organism. Such success was dependent on exploiting knowledge of the epidemiology of the disease in the natural setting.

With the availability of effective vaccines and therapeutics, perhaps practitioners have become too reliant on disease control that comes in a bottle as opposed to concentrating on the other components of disease control. Areas that must be considered include the health status of animal introductions (temporary or permanent); the quality of feed; the quality of animal drinking water; the risk posed by exposure to wildlife; the risk posed by caretakers, service providers, and visitors; the risk posed by arthropods; the role equipment may play in the introduction or spread of disease agents; and the risk of wind-delivered pathogens.

Table 1
Biosecurity as a risk-analysis activity

Step	Focus
Risk assessment	What are the disease problems of concern?
	How large are the problems (effect)?
	How likely are they to occur?
Risk management	Methods of prevention
Risk communication	Production team (all levels)
	Suppliers
	Customers

The development of a biosecurity plan for a cattle operation can be likened to HACCP or a risk-analysis activity (Table 1). Development of the plan should commence with a risk assessment in which the problems or agents of concern are identified, their likely effect is quantified, and the likelihood of their introduction is estimated. Based on this exercise, a prioritized list can be made for the disease agents of most interest. Subsequently, a targeted risk management plan can be developed for those agents of highest priority. The success of the plan can be ensured only if there is adequate risk communication activity. Risk communication includes communicating the management plan to all levels of the production team and to the suppliers and the customers. The production team has an obvious role in carrying out the biosecurity activities and in communicating any changes to the plan that are needed. Suppliers of feed and other products must be partners in the management plan so that disease agents are not inadvertently introduced with inputs to the operation. Customers can be partners in the biosecurity plan in that there may be marketing advantages for the animals or products produced under a good biosecurity plan. The operation supplying the animals becomes the source (supplier) for the next phase of the chain, whether the product is in the form of seedstock or replacements or even food and other products.

Clearly, the biosecurity plan must be individualized for each operation. Each operator has a different set of concerns and different perceptions of risk. Each individual production unit also has its own windows of vulnerability. The following articles in this issue of the *Veterinary Clinics of North America: Food Animal Practice* present a few of the concepts to be considered in developing a biosecurity plan based on the body system and age of the animal or means of disease agent transmission. Certain articles are meant to present some of the overarching principles of a biosecurity plan.

References

[1] American Society for Microbiology Task Force. Report of the American Society for Microbiology task force on antibiotic resistance. Washington, DC: American Society for Microbiology; 1995.

[2] American Veterinary Medical Association. AVMA judicious therapeutic use of antimicro-bials. Available at: http://www.avma.org/onlnews/javma/jan99/s011599b.htm. Accessed October 5, 2001.

[3] Anderson JF. Biosecurity—a new term for an old concept: how to apply it. Bovine Prac-titioner 1998;32:61–70.

[4] Cohen M. Epidemiology of drug resistance: implications of a post-antimicrobial era. Science 1992;257:1050–5.

[5] Harrison PF, Lederberg J. Antimicrobial resistance: issues and options, workshop report. Washington, DC: Institute of Medicine, National Academy Press; 1998. p. 1–115.

[6] Martin SW, Meek AH, Willeberg P. Veterinary epidemiology. Ames (IA): Iowa State University Press 1987. p. 15.

[7] Thomson JU. Biosecurity: preventing and controlling diseases in the beef herd. In: Pro-ceedings of the Annual Meeting of the Livestock Conservation Institute. Nashville (TN); 1999. p. 49–51.

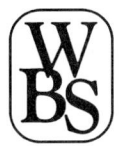

THE VETERINARY
CLINICS
Food Animal
Practice

Vet Clin Food Anim 18 (2002) 7–34

Biosecurity for neonatal gastrointestinal diseases

George M.Barrington, DVM, PhD*, John M. Gay,
DVM, PhD, James F. Evermann, MS, PhD

*Department of Veterinary Clinical Sciences, College of Veterinary Medicine,
Washington State University, Pullman, WA 99164, USA*

Calves are born and raised in a wide diversity of environments and housing conditions, all of which affect the risk of neonatal enteric infectious disease. At one extreme are calves born in closed-beef cow–calf operations under low-density conditions on open range, such as in the low-rainfall areas of the Intermountain United States. This environment closely resembles the conditions in which the infectious agents and their hosts co-evolved before domestication. In this setting, the risk of introducing new strains of infectious agents is low, direct contact among calves is minimized, the opportunity for transmission by people and equipment is minimal, and fecal material is dispersed and exposed to environmental factors (i.e., insects, desiccation, and ultraviolet radiation) that inactivate most microorganisms. At the other exposure extreme, calves are raised in enclosed housing on continuous-flow, custom calf-raising operations. In this environment, calves are assembled from multiple herds and from sales channels in which the risk of heavy exposure to a variety of infectious agents is high. Calves are often in direct contact with one another, the physical space per calf is limited, and the risk of transmission by people and equipment is high. If housed, ventilation is often inadequate, resulting in a high relative humidity; fecal material is concentrated, with a high moisture content and without full exposure to direct sunlight. Vermin such as flies and rodents are often present in high numbers, and nutrition is provided by assembled feedstuffs of varying quality and nutritional value rather than from dam's milk. Between these two extremes are calves raised in individual hutches on dairies of their origin or beef calves raised in intensively managed rotational grazing systems in high-rainfall areas.

---

* Corresponding author.
E-mail address: geob@vetmed.wsu.edu (G.M. Barrington).

Diarrhea is the most important disease of neonatal calves and results in the greatest economic loss due to disease in this age group in both dairy and beef calves [25]. Earlier studies conducted by the US Department of Agriculture found that enteric pathogens are associated with the death of up to 25% of the US calf crop annually [43]. More recently, a retrospective survey of dairy producers found that 52% (standard error [SE] ± 2.6%) of total death losses in preweaned heifers were caused by diarrhea [65]. In beef calves, the percentage of calves from birth to 21 days of age dying from diarrhea was 5.5% (SE ± 1.3%) [10]. Neonatal calf diarrhea is a complex, multifactorial condition with numerous factors, including pathogen exposure, strain variation, environmental conditions, management conditions, nutritional state, and immune status all interacting to cause loss in preweaned beef and dairy calves. Most, if not all, of these factors are related to biosecurity in beef and dairy calf-raising practices. Many are under management control, and most are not specific to a single infectious agent. Biosecurity is not a new concept in animal agriculture; rather, it is largely a redefinition of earlier ideas and practices historically considered to be good animal husbandry. This observation is evident when one notices in early veterinary textbooks the calls for cleanliness, disinfection, and isolation of herd replacements and sick animals [4].

General epidemiologic concepts

The two major thrusts of infectious disease biosecurity are (1) reducing the likelihood of introduction of an infectious agent into a group (external biosecurity) and (2) reducing the likelihood of its transmission when present (internal or within-herd biosecurity, or biocontainment). When approaching the control and prevention of neonatal enteric infections, knowledge of several general infectious disease epidemiology principles is useful. Essential information for designing a herd-specific control program for any infectious disease includes (1) the reservoir, (2) the modes of transmission and the agent characteristics related to each, (3) the incubation period, and (4) the period of communicability. The minimum incubation period (along with the infectious dose and the age of the calf) is critical because, for example, it establishes the maximum length of time a susceptible calf can be present in a critical calving facility before it could begin to contaminate the area if it were infected at birth. The most important reservoir for these enteric agents is previously or currently infected cattle, which is critical for producers to recognize when they are considering purchasing animals and when they are managing contact between different age groups within a herd.

Most of these agents transmit predominately by the fecal-oral route from the feces of infected animals to the mouths of susceptible animals, and do so efficiently. Immediate transmission occurs when infected animals are housed with susceptible animals in conditions that allow nose-to-nose contact or inhalation of aerosols produced by coughing, urinating, or defecating.

Indirect contact transmission requires that the infectious agent survive in the environment. Most agents of neonatal calf diarrhea survive well in nearly all environmental conditions, remaining in the environment where they can be transmitted indirectly by contact with contaminated feces, fomites such as equipment, or mechanical vectors such as flies. For enteric agents transmitted by indirect contact, key factors include the number of organisms shed in the feces and their survival characteristics in the environment compared with the infectious dose required to initiate infection in susceptible hosts. Information on the environmental survival characteristics of an indirectly transmitted agent is needed to determine how long that agent is likely to remain at an infectious dose once the area is contaminated with it. All of this is critical information for determining how to manage livestock flow through an existing set of facilities and to otherwise minimize disease transmission through management practices. The relationship between infecting agents and the environment is complex, involving factors such as the physical characteristics of the substrate material (e.g., feces, water, milk, manure slurry, dust), temperature, pH, water activity, and competing microorganisms. As a consequence, these relationships are not well defined for many combinations encountered in the farm environment.

With the rare exception, it is likely that most infectious enteric agents of cattle co-evolved with their bovine hosts long before their domestication thousands of years ago [51,52]. If an agent was able to survive under the free-range conditions of the wild bovine, it is likely that transmission occurs relatively easily in the environment of the intensively managed domesticated bovine of today. Indeed, these agents are shed by infected animals in numbers several logarithms higher per gram of feces than the total number required to infect the typical susceptible calf. Additionally, these agents have been shown to be extraordinarily flexible with regard to their genetic make-up and through survival of the fittest can rapidly take advantage of new environments and management systems. Consequently, intervention strategies devoted to a single control point may be successful in the short run but are likely to prove unsuccessful over the long run.

An important concept that is often overlooked, particularly in the midst of clinical disease outbreaks, is the "iceberg principle." This concept is in effect both within and between herds. Between herds, clinical disease is normally seen in only a minority of herds, in which its occurrence implies significant, suboptimal management conditions. Within herds, generally only a small proportion of affected animals are clinically affected, with most being subclinically infected. For most diseases, both infectious and noninfectious, the ratio between clinical cases and subclinical cases is typically 1:5 to 1:20. In some circumstances, a herd can be widely infected with an agent, yet few if any clinical cases occur. Consideration of the iceberg principle helps prioritize efforts because in most outbreaks, attention is typically but erroneously focused only on individual animals displaying clinical signs. To wit, if isolation and sanitation practices are to be an important component of a disease control strategy, the iceberg principle suggests that to be effective, such measures must be applied to all exposed animals and not just those that exhibit clinical signs.

General cleaning and disinfection considerations

Appropriate cleaning and disinfection procedures are critical to breaking fecal-oral transmission cycles of enteric agents that contaminate housing, feeding, or treatment equipment or other vectors and fomites. Because personal hygiene is crucial to stopping the transmission of these agents in the human hospital environment, it is also a critical component in the intense livestock production environment as well. This personal hygiene includes frequent, effective hand washing of sufficient duration with soap followed by an alcohol-based hand disinfectant [50], cleaning and disinfecting boots, and washing work clothes with bleach followed by hot air drying. Cleaning and disinfection procedures are not without pitfalls, however, and adherence to a sound protocol covering all of the infectious agents of concern is critical for long-term success. Procedures that do not affect a resistant agent such as *Cryptosporidia* oocysts or rotavirus may spread it from areas of high concentration across previously uncontaminated surfaces, where it can then contaminate materials such as water and feed at sufficient levels to provide an infectious dose. The most important first step is thorough cleaning to remove organic material (e.g., feces, milk film) before applying disinfectant [46]. Vigorous cleaning (scraping, scrubbing, flushing) cannot be replaced by applying disinfectants in larger quantities or with higher pressure. For any protocol or in nature, destruction of microorganisms initially follows a first-order logarithmic decay process and then slows [74]. In relation to the amount of time required to destroy one half of the initial population, approximately three time periods are required for a one-logarithmic (90%) reduction, six for a two-logarithmic (99%) reduction, nine for a three-logarithmic (99.9%) reduction, and so on. In addition to contact time, the concentration, temperature, pH, water content, water hardness, and amount of organic material present are critical variables determining the success of chemical disinfection. Importantly, the relationships between these factors are not straightforward [54]. For example, halving the concentration of formaldehyde requires a 2-fold increase in contact time to obtain similar microbial destruction, whereas halving the concentration of phenolics requires a 64-fold increase in contact time. A 10°C rise in temperature increases the activity of alcohols 30-fold, yet increases the activity of formaldehyde only 1.5-fold. Iodophors are highly active at low pH but are inactive at an alkaline pH. In general, effectively applied live steam inactivates the broadest range of microorganisms.

Sodium hypochlorite (bleach, NaOCl) at a sufficient concentration, contact time, and temperature combination is effective against the bacterial and viral agents of neonatal enteric disease [87], but at practical levels is not effective against *Cryptosporidium* oocysts. It is readily available as 5.25% (household bleach) and 12.75% solutions, and it is cost effective and environmentally safe. Because it begins dissipating on dilution, however, the Centers for Disease Control recommends that diluted solutions should be used within 24 hours and that they should be stored in opaque containers. Sodium hypochlorite is rapidly inactivated by the presence of any appreciable organic material; for example, 1% albumin reduces its effectiveness by six logs, and increasing concentration or contact time does not recover this loss. Bacteria in biofilms are 150 to 3000 times more resistant. In solution, hypochlorus acid is the active form of the free chlorine. It is most available at a pH level of 6, dropping to 80% of the free chlorine at pH 7 and to 25% at pH 8, suggesting that the pH of disinfectant solutions should be monitored regularly as part of disinfection protocols. Below pH 6, it is more corrosive to metals, and more chlorine gas is released. Testing kits can be used to monitor free chlorine as part of disinfection protocols; however, because these kits measure both hypochlorus acid and hypochlorite ion (nonactive form), pH must also be considered. Recommended concentrations for use in human environments range from 500 ppm (1:100 dilution of 5.25% household bleach) and 10-minute contact time at room temperature to 5000 ppm (1:10 dilution of 5.25% bleach) and 1-minute contact time at room temperature, the higher concentrations being used in more critical areas. For viruses in veterinary hospitals and kennels, a recommended dilution of household bleach is 1:32, which results in a 0.175% sodium hypochlorite solution and a 10-minute contact time at room temperature [93] at pH 6 to 7.

The characteristics of environmental surfaces targeted for disinfection in the farm environment also influence the success or failure of various procedures [62]. For example, unfinished plywood retains 15-fold more microorganisms than varnished plywood, which supports 15-fold more microorganisms than plastic surfaces. On smooth, ideal surfaces physical removal of visible contamination by thorough washing with soap and water removes 99% of the microbial load (two logs). On typical housing surfaces, however, washing only removes 90% (one log). Proper disinfection removes an additional 6% to 7%, and terminal fumigation removes 1% to 2%. Disinfection after washing is an important step, particularly if the surface remains damp, because remaining bacteria can proliferate in the minimal nutrients leaching from wet wood and because washing can disperse an infectious agent from limited areas of high concentration broadly across other surfaces. The application of high-pressure sprays can aerosolize organisms, allowing dissemination to distant sites and posing a risk to operators if zoonotic organisms are present.

Gastrointestinal pathogens of concern

The most frequently recognized agents causing neonatal calf diarrhea include *Escherichia coli (E. coli)* spp., rotavirus, coronavirus, cryptosporidia, coccidia, and *Salmonella* spp [1,85,96,102]. With the exception of *Salmonella* spp. and specific strains of *E. coli*, these organisms are ubiquitous and holoendemic, being present within the gastrointestinal tract of some if not most healthy, mature cattle, albeit in low concentrations and without clinical signs of infection. Because most all cattle are exposed to these agents at some point in their life if not continuously, they must therefore develop active immunity against these organisms. Undoubtedly, most animals develop active immunity to these organisms after infection by natural exposure to low infective doses shed by subclinically infected herd mates. Ideally, such infections result in the stimulation of immunity without the development of adverse or serious clinical disease. Alternatively, active immunity can also be developed by successful immunization with antigenically similar strains.

Mixed infections with these agents are a common phenomenon during calfhood. Management practices that minimize the risk of clinical disease by one organism generally reduce the risk of clinical disease by others. In a study of 59 calves younger than 3 weeks old from 12 beef and dairy herds with calf-scour problems, Moon and coworkers [61] found that "most infections were mixed and diarrheal calves from the same herd frequently had different infections." In a survey of 490 preweaned calves from 45 calf-scour outbreaks, Reynolds et al [85] found that 29% of the clinical infections were mixed. Similarly, Snodgrass and coworkers [96] found that 21% of diarrheic calves less than 1 month old on 32 beef and dairy farms had mixed infections. Finally, in a study of 218 diarrheic calves less than 1 month old from 65 dairy herds, 25% of calves had mixed infections consisting primarily of rotavirus and *Cryptosporidium parvum* [33]. In most of these surveys, the most prevalent agent in diarrheic calves is rotavirus, the second being *C. parvum* at approximately half the prevalence of rotavirus. In surveys that included clinically normal herd mates, similar profiles of infectious agents were also found in the feces of these animals but at lower prevalences. These findings suggest that enteric pathogens of calves function more as secondary opportunists than as highly virulent primary pathogens. The occurrence of clinical disease therefore suggests that weaknesses are present in calf management and husbandry on those premises. Because nearly all of these pathogens are already present on most operations, control of enteric disease must therefore be focused on the interfaces between individual animals and groups of animals rather than on preventing their arrival on the operation, the traditional focus of most biosecurity efforts.

Numerous other pathogens have been implicated in neonatal diarrhea, including *Campylobacter* spp., *Clostridium* spp., Parvovirus, Breda virus, and bovine viral diarrhea virus; however, their importance in field outbreaks of diarrhea is currently unknown. Regardless, practices that are sufficient to control the common enteric agents likely will also control the lesser-known agents as well.

Salmonella

Subsets of *Salmonella enterica* serovars, such as *S.* Typhimurium and *S.* Dublin, are important causes of diarrhea in dairy and veal calves, whereas infections in single-suckle beef calves are infrequent. The pathophysiology of enteric salmonella infections is complex, involving inflammation and necrosis, increased fluid secretion and decreased absorption and digestion. In addition to enteric manifestations of disease, infected calves are frequently septicemic, which results in more severe clinical signs. Bacteremia is common in calves less than 1 month of age and is often manifested systemically as polyarthritis, meningitis, or uveitis. In addition to shedding the agent in their feces, calves developing septicemia often shed the agent in their urine and oronasal secretions even before the onset of clinical signs. The lack of awareness about the potential for shedding from the oronasal area is particularly dangerous because this source leads to spread through contamination of feeding and treatment utensils and hands, severely compromising internal biosecurity programs. Hardman and coworkers [38] found that in natural outbreaks of individually penned calves, approximately 60% of transmission was by direct contact, whereas 40% was by indirect routes, including aerosols, fomites, and vectors. This finding suggests that emphasis should be placed more broadly on controlling all means of transmission, including aerosols [105].

Salmonella spp. are hardy organisms that are well adapted to surviving in the environment [31]. They are able to proliferate rapidly at high ambient temperatures in waste milk, colostrum, and moist feeds. In the absence of direct sunlight or predation by other microorganisms, *Salmonella* spp. can survive in wet or dry substrates or on surfaces for years, particularly if they are protected by biological films such as dried saliva, milk, or fat. Biological films also protect organisms from the action of chemical disinfectants. In an experiment that simulated a barn floor under defecating cows, *Salmonella* spp. were shown to survive for 5.5 years [72]. These researchers also found *S.* Typhimurium in an empty slurry pit that had not been used for 4 years. Because *Salmonella* spp. that infect cattle can infect and proliferate in the intestinal tracts of most other animals in a farm environment (including other livestock, humans, domestic pets, rodents, and birds), these other species may also be involved in disease transmission. For example, allowing cats access to stored feeds has been identified as a risk factor for salmonella outbreaks [26]. Serotypes that frequently infect cattle are typically introduced into a herd by subclinical or incubating carrier animals and only occasionally in feedstuffs. Many of the other serotypes imported onto farms in purchased feedstuffs appear unable to establish viable transmission cycles between cattle, instead causing only sporadic infections.

Of special note is that *Salmonella* spp. and *C. parvum* infections in livestock present significant zoonotic disease risks to in-contact people and in turn to their contacts, particularly young children, the elderly, and the immunocompromised. Because of these significant health risks, indirect and direct contact between susceptible individuals and livestock potentially infected with these agents should be minimized. Hands should be washed well, using soap and warm water and scrubbing for 15 seconds followed by an alcohol-based antiseptic hand rub [50] before eating or returning to the household. Inhalation of potentially contaminated dusts or aerosols, particularly those generated by cleaning procedures such as high-pressure washing, should be minimized. To reduce the likelihood of introducing these agents into the household and their transmission to susceptible humans or domestic pets, equipment, outer garments, and footwear exposed to potentially infected animals and their discharges should not be brought into the household.

Escherichia coli

As a major bacterial component of feces from warm-blooded animals, *E. coli* are ubiquitous in the environment of neonatal beef and dairy calves. All *E. coli* types can cause colisepticemia, but relatively few can cause enteric disease. Enteric *E. coli* infections are classified into several forms, including enterotoxigenic, enteropathogenic, enteroinvasive, enterohemorrhagic, and enteroadherent [53]. Enterotoxigenic *E. coli* are the most common form associated with disease in calves. The ability of enterotoxigenic *E. coli* to cause severe herd outbreaks of diarrhea in calves results from the expression of virulence factors, including adhesins (pili, fimbria) and enterotoxins. Adhesins (e.g., K99, F41, K88) are surface molecules that enable the bacteria to attach to specific receptors located on the intestinal epithelium of calves less than 3 days old. Once attached to intestinal cells via adhesins, bacterial expression of enterotoxins triggers intestinal fluid secretion in excess of absorptive capacity. In addition to enteric diseases caused by *E. coli*, systemic invasion by certain strains can result in septic shock and low-grade diarrhea. Diarrhea observed in these calves is generally thought to be due to endotoxemia secondary to bacteremia rather than production of enterotoxins.

Although not as hardy as *Salmonella* spp., *E. coli* survive well on typical farm environmental surfaces and in feces and dust protected from moisture and direct sunlight [8,58]. In experimentally inoculated cow manure or fresh slurry under common farm environmental conditions, both organisms decrease by one log in 1 to 3 weeks [42]. Depending on the surface characteristics, the numbers of organisms decline at about 0.25 log per day. Generally, the rate of decline is slower at lower humidity, but proliferation can occur on surfaces under saturated conditions with minimal organic nutrients (0.5 mg/L). Exposure to ultraviolet components in direct sunlight rapidly kills the organism [24].

Rotavirus

Rotavirus is a double-stranded, nonenveloped RNA virus. Rotaviruses are the most common cause of bovine neonatal diarrhea, the incidence of infection often approaching 100% in herds, and up to one half of infections resulting in clinical disease. Infection usually occurs between 4 and 14 days of age, although younger and older calves can be affected [66]. Because the median infectious dose for rotaviral infections in other species is 10 infectious particles or less [36,103], the infectious dose for neonatal calves is likely similar. Viral invasion of small intestinal villus epithelium occurs through the luminal surface, resulting in cell destruction and shedding of damaged cells into the intestinal lumen. As a consequence of this infection route, the incubation period is short, and large numbers of virus particles are produced rapidly. Within 48 hours of initial infection, the virus can reach 1×10^{10} (ten billion) virus particles per gram of feces. Villous atrophy and cellular damage result in maldigestion and malabsorption. Maldigestion results from the loss of hydrolytic enzymes produced by mature villous cells. Failure to hydrolyze milk lactose results in lactose transit into the large intestine, where it acts osmotically, pulling water into the intestinal lumen. In addition to decreased enzyme activity, sodium and water transport processes are impaired, resulting in malabsorption. Some rotavirus strains are pneumotropic, replicating in the respiratory tract and transmitting via inhalation and by the fecal-oral route. Rotavirus is carried in adult cattle through nonclinical infection with intermittent fecal shedding [47]. Shedding increases coincident with later stages of gestation and for up to 4 weeks postpartum. In some management situations, this maternal shedding may account for most virus exposures to neonatal calves [28].

Being a nonenveloped RNA virus, rotavirus is relatively stable in the environment, being infectious in feces for up to 6 months at 25°C. In smears of human feces, human rotavirus was more stable at lower temperatures and at humidity extremes [59]. Infectious particles declined by 1 log in 29 days at 4°C and 93% relative humidity, in 16 days at 4°C and 13% relative humidity, in 2.2 days at 20°C and 55% relative humidity, and in 1.5 days at 37°C and 13% relative humidity. Some research suggests that bovine rotavirus may be more resistant than human rotavirus. Virus stability in water varies with water quality and temperature, ranging from being very stable in clean water at 4°C to falling 2 logs in 10 days in typical river water at 20°C [84]. As temperatures above 60°C are lethal to the virus [68], standard milk pasteurization procedures are effective against it. Rotavirus is susceptible to sufficient concentrations of sodium hypochlorite (1750 ppm) but is relatively resistant to many common disinfectants, such as chlorhexidine, under the same exposure conditions. Because as a nonenveloped virus it is not affected by soaps, washing with soap alone may actually spread the virus around on the washed surface [23].

Coronavirus

Coronavirus is an enveloped single-stranded RNA virus and is not as stable in the environment as rotavirus [27]. Serologic studies have demonstrated that the prevalence of serum antibodies to coronavirus approaches

100% in adult beef and dairy cattle. Calves are typically infected by corona-virus between 4 and 30 days of life [66]. Although they may not be the same virus strains, evidence is mounting that a respiratory form as well as the enteric form occurs [97]. Similar to rotavirus, infection results in damage to intestinal villous epithelium; however, infection by coronavirus often results in more severe disease manifestations because the degree of villous atrophy is greater and both the large and small intestines are affected. As described for rotavirus, coronavirus is carried in adult cattle through noncli-nical infection and is shed in fecal matter. Because of their envelope, these viruses retain infectiousness better at lower rather than higher relative humidity [24] and are considerably more sensitive to soaps and common dis-infectants than are nonenveloped viruses. This virus is more active in the colder climates and has been reported to cause winter dysentery in adult cattle [16,27]. Control of coronavirus (and rotavirus) infections in calves relies on continual presence of a protective antibody within the gut lumen, which can be achieved by allowing neonates to ingest colostrum or milk containing these specific antibodies from their dams (lactogenic immunity) [19].

Cryptosporidia

Cryptosporidium parvum is a common cause of neonatal calf diarrhea between 7 and 21 days of age, rarely causing diarrhea at less than 7 or more than 28 days of age [22]. Similar to rotavirus and coronavirus infection, the incidence of infection with cryptosporidia often approaches 100% in the first month of life, infection often occurs concurrently with rotavirus and coro-navirus infections, and a respiratory form may occur. Unlike most other enteric protozoa, *Cryptosporidium* are immediately infectious when passed and can infect other susceptible hosts through direct contact. Because *Cryptosporidium* can autoinfect the original host, the infectious dose can be exceedingly small. For example, the median infectious dose for humans is only 87 oocysts [29], and some researchers suggest it is even lower for neo-natal calves. Cryptosporidia infect and invade enterocytes in the distal small intestine, causing villous atrophy and fusion that result in malabsorption and maldigestion. Infected calves may shed 10^5 to 10^7 oocysts per gram of feces beginning with the onset of clinical signs. Importantly, fecal shedding can continue days after clinical signs subside. In California beef cow–calf herds, Atwill et al [7] found that higher stocking densities, longer calving periods, and wetter seasons were associated with higher fecal shedding pre-valences in calves. Research findings on the adult carrier state are conflict-ing, because some have found that adult carrier animals are common [92], whereas others have found that few if any asymptomatic adult cattle appar-ently shed *Cryptosporidium parvum* in appreciable numbers [6,55]. Undoubt-edly, infected calves are likely the most important reservoir for continuing the fecal-oral cycle on most farms because of the large numbers of oocysts that they excrete in close proximity to susceptible calves [22].

In the environment, cryptosporidia are extremely resistant to most veterinary disinfectants except 5% ammonia, 6% hydrogen peroxide, or 10% formalin [14,86,107]. They survive well in water, requiring 4 to 11 weeks to decline by 1 log [15]. Because the oocysts adhere in large numbers to the plastic and rubber surfaces of common calf-feeding and treatment equipment such as nipples, bottles, and buckets (E.R. Atwill, DVM, PhD, 2001, personal communication), common sanitation procedures are not likely to prevent fomite transmission by these items. A portion of the oocysts still retain their infectivity after mild freezing [30]. On the other hand, complete drying in thin, naturally infected fecal smears on wood kills the oocysts within 1 to 4 days [2]. Finally, because moist heating at 45°C for 20 minutes kills the oocysts [3], standard pasteurization procedures (e.g., 63°C for 30 minutes, 72°C for 15 seconds) are effective.

Coccidia

Eimeria bovis and *E. zurnii* are the species of coccidia most commonly associated with calf diarrhea. With a prepatent period of approximately 17 days, calves exposed to an infectious dose shortly after birth can present with bloody diarrhea and anemia by the third week of life. Diagnosis is easiest in calves with acute infections because many shed large numbers of oocysts in the feces. Chronically infected calves may only shed small to moderate numbers of oocysts in the stool, however, making diagnosis more difficult.

Risk factors related to spread of gastrointestinal pathogens

A large number of risk factors are potentially associated with the development of neonatal calf diarrhea. These factors can be categorized into those that are related to either (1) the calf, (2) the infectious agent, or (3) the environment of the calf. Recognizing the presence of specific risk factors on the premises followed by interpreting the relative significance of each factor is required for the implementation and coordination of specific biosecurity practices to mitigate the problem of enteric disease on that farm. Although Pence et al [70] do not provide any information on validation, they do provide a risk assessment-scoring sheet for neonatal diarrhea in beef herds. On most operations, the presence and importance of these risk factors change over time, sometimes quite suddenly, as sources of animals, husbandry practices, and, to a lesser degree, physical facilities often change with turnover of employees and in response to changes in economic conditions.

Risk factors associated with the calf

The presence of developmental, congenital, or heritable abnormalities in a calf can be a risk factor depending on the character, location, and degree of the defect. Certainly any abnormality that prevents a calf from functioning normally (e.g., ambulating or obtaining adequate nutrition) can increase the chance of a severe enteric infection.

Failure of passive transfer of maternal immunity through colostrum ingestion is a major risk factor for development of neonatal diarrhea [21,56]. In the 1992 US Department of Agriculture National Dairy Heifer Evaluation Project, Wells et al [108] found that feeding a sufficient amount of colostrum soon enough after birth prevented 31% of the dairy heifer mortality that occurred in the first 21 days of life. Colostrum provides the necessary components of immunity during the time when a calf is immunonaive yet exposed to pathogens in its environment. Consumption of colostral immunoglobulin from resident cows in a herd is likely to provide immunologic protection specific to the strains of pathogens found within that herd. Importantly, even if colostral immunoglobulin specificity is appropriate for specific pathogens, maximum protection is ultimately dependent on the ingestion and absorption of an adequate mass of immunoglobulin by the calf. Immunoglobulin concentration varies from breed to breed, however, as well as from cow to cow within a breed. Such differences are well illustrated by the fact that the average concentration of immunoglobulin in beef cow colostrum is 2 to 3 times greater than that of dairy cow colostrum [73,106]. As expected, the most important factor involved in failure of passive transfer in dairy calves is low immunoglobulin–concentration colostrum, whereas in beef calves delayed suckling is a leading cause [12]. For dairy cows, colostrum that is not from first milking, from cows that leaked milk, or from cows that weighed more than 20 lb should not be used for passive transfer [73]. In certain situations, beef calves may be provided alternate sources of colostrum, including colostrum obtained from nearby dairies. Again, it is imperative to appreciate that because the average immunoglobulin concentration of dairy cow colostrum is low compared with beef cow colostrum, an adequate volume (4 L) of appropriately selected dairy cow colostrum must be fed. In addition, one must also consider the risk of introducing novel pathogens when supplementing calves with an off-farm source of nonpasteurized colostrum. Unless properly pasteurized, dairy colostrum purchased for administration to beef calves in place of their dam's colostrum may be contaminated with infectious doses of undesirable infectious agents such as *Mycobacterium avium* subsp. *paratuberculosis* as well as the enteric agents of concern described in this article.

The nutritional status of the dam (particularly during late gestation, when the fetus is active metabolically and growing exponentially) is often of concern in relation to the immune status and health of the calf after birth [21]. The effect of nutrition and other factors such as dystocia on passive transfer in dairy cattle was recently reviewed by Quigley and Drewry [75]. There is little evidence of a direct link between gestational cow nutrition and immunoglobulin concentration of the calves [71]. The weak calf syndrome, however, has been reported in beef cattle when prepartum cows consuming diets deficient in protein or energy (protein-energy malnutrition), either because of improper feeding practices or other factors such as severe weather events, in late gestation subsequently calve in environments in which the temperature is below the thermoneutral zone of the calf [67,69]. Therefore, it is only logical to recommend that producers provide feeds adequate in quantity and quality to meet National Research Council requirements for beef cattle and dairy cattle during gestation and lactation.

In comparison with beef calves, dairy calves are often fed milk replacer diets because the cost is lower than that of cows' milk. The composition and quality of milk replacers varies considerably, however, much to the detriment of very young calves with limited digestive capabilities. Some milk replacers contain heat-denatured, milk-origin proteins, poorly digestible vegetable-origin proteins, or nonlactose carbohydrate sources that the intestinal enzymes of neonatal calves cannot digest. Consumption of such products frequently results in inadequate nutrition, poor growth rates, and high morbidity and mortality due to enteric diseases [83]. Often the feeding recommendations for even high-quality milk replacers are designed for 60-lb calves, rather than the average 90-lb Holstein calf, placing the larger calves into a negative energy and protein balance until their starter consumption increases sufficiently. Nutrition of the neonatal calf is an active area of research, much of which has been summarized by Davis and Drackley [21], and changes in nutritional guidelines often reduce the risk of neonatal disease. In addition, excellent reviews on the relationship between neonatal digestive physiology and the different ingredients contained in milk replacers are available [37,82].

If nonsaleable milk is fed, it should be pasteurized before feeding to reduce the likelihood of transmitting these and other infectious enteric agents. A recent study found that raw milk and mixed milk replacer often contain high numbers of bacteria, ranging from 10^3 colony-forming units (CFUs)/mL for mixed milk replacer to more than 10^6 CFUs/mL for hospital milk [94]. Another study found that calves fed pasteurized waste milk perform better in terms of weight gain, mortality, morbidity, and health costs than those fed the same milk raw, even in the absence of the specific enteric agents of concern discussed in this article [45]. Pasteurization controls their milk-borne transmission as well.

Finally, the source of calves is a risk factor for enteric diseases when calves have been commingled from several sources or origins. Certainly, calves purchased from sale yards are more likely to have been exposed to higher concentrations and to a wider variety of pathogens compared with single-source calves or calves on pasture. Frequently, calves are purchased from market sources to graft onto cows that have lost their own offspring. Such purchased calves often introduce new strains of infectious agents that then spread through the herd in an outbreak fashion, making the situation considerably worse. In addition to increased exposure to pathogens, calves transiting through sale yards are likely to be under more severe physiologic stress and more likely to have had failure of passive transfer [106]. A study of beef cow–calf herds found that purchasing such calves at less than 4 weeks of age increased the likelihood of a high-mortality diarrhea outbreak over four-fold [91].

Risk factors associated with the infectious agent

The primary risk factors associated with infectious agents that cause enteric infections include specific virulence factors, the size of the inoculum or pathogen load, and whether single or multiple infections exist.

As mentioned previously, virulence factors associated with bacteria include structural elements such as pili that allow bacteria to attach to the host, as well as bacterial products that augment bacterial cell growth, enhance host cell damage, or negate the immune response of the host. Both exotoxins and endotoxins can have adverse effects. Other virulence factors of enteric bacteria include those that enhance bacterial ability to resist antimicrobial agents through expression of drug resistance plasmids or integrons.

Virulence factors associated with enteric viruses or protozoa are less well described. Different strains or serotypes of viruses have been identified; however, most strains of a particular virus appear to act similarly. The challenge load of enteric bacteria, protozoa, and viruses from periparturient cattle is high because of the aforementioned physiologic immunosuppression [28].

When considering biosecurity or biocontainment, it is critical to realize that the size of the inoculum or the pathogen concentration (exposure dose) is a major factor in determining the degree of clinical disease and the rapidity of its onset rather than whether exposure occurs. This is especially true when considering the ubiquitous agents involved in bovine neonatal diarrhea, because none are extraordinarily virulent in their own right. It is logical to conclude that a large enough exposure dose, such as that likely to occur during outbreaks, will undoubtedly overwhelm even the best passive transfer of immunity and lead to an expanding outbreak in previously unaffected calves.

Risk factors associated with the environment of the calf

Risk factors for neonatal diarrhea associated with the environment of the calf are likely to be the most amenable to the implementation of specific biosecurity measures. Specific risk factors include the atmospheric conditions (temperature, humidity, wind chill, ventilation, air quality, and so forth); housing (individual calf hutches, enclosed group pens, dispersal on pasture); the physical environment (calving area, bedding, other animals, cleaning protocols, and so forth); stocking density; general hygiene and hygiene related to feeding practices; and miscellaneous stresses due to handling, surgery transportation, and the like.

Many of these potential risk factors are under management control. Because of the difficulty of executing rigorously designed large-scale studies with sufficient herd numbers to evaluate all potential risk factors, reasoning from biological plausibility is often the only basis for developing interventions when sufficient evidence is not available. Although some findings are conflicting, a limited number of field studies of different size and rigor do provide guidance for some of these risk factors. For example, Bendali et al [11] found that cleaning of the calving area immediately before calving was associated with an increased risk of neonatal diarrhea in beef calves compared with not cleaning it, whereas cleaning it after calving was associated with a decreased risk. They also found that greater cow cleanliness was associated with decreased risk. Based on data from the 1997 US Department of Agriculture National Beef Cow-Calf Study, Sanderson and Dargatz [88] reported that although 41% of birth-to-weaning mortality was attributable to dystocia, 11% was due to confined calving. In the 1992 US Department of Agriculture National Dairy Heifer Evaluation Project, Wells et al [108] found that separating heifers from their dams within the first 24 hours after birth prevented 16% of the dairy heifer mortality that occurred during the first 21 days of life. Quigely et al [76] found that calves administered sufficient amounts of colostrum and housed in individual calf hutches shed fewer enteric pathogens in their feces than calves left to nurse their dam and housed in an enclosed space with mechanical ventilation. Schumann et al [91] found that increased risk of neonatal diarrhea in beef calves was associated with wintering cows and primigravida heifers together, providing limited shelter to nursing pairs, and an increased percentage of poorly drained ground in the nursing area. Although the occurrence of diarrhea was not affected, Sivula et al [95] found that increased gain was associated with all-in, all-out group management of weaned dairy calves.

Sufficient ventilation is important to the health of housed calves [5,104]. Besides being critical for removal of transpired water vapor and reducing humidity, sufficient ventilation in enclosed housing also removes infectious aerosols. Reducing humidity can also reduce the survival time of aerosolized and surface-borne infectious agents. Although more important for respiratory disease, these factors in turn have an effect on the risk of enteric disease. Because salmonellosis, cryptosporidiosis, rotavirus, and coronavirus agents can be transmitted by aerosols, procedures that produce aerosols (pressure washing, housing flush systems) considerably increase the risk of transmission [9]. For example, Mohammed et al [60] found that dairy calves raised outside or in mechanically ventilated buildings were five-fold less likely to shed *Cryptosporidia parvum* oocysts than those raised in nonventilated barns.

Importance of other animate vectors

Within the calf's environment, other animal species may function as mechanical or biological vectors of enteric infectious agents, particularly if they are present in large numbers and no control efforts are in effect. These species include domestic pets, humans, and vermin such as insects, rodents, and birds.

One of the most overlooked vectors that presents a significant disease transmission risk is the nuisance fly, particularly the house fly, *Musca domestica* [35]. During summer months before severe frosts, fly populations typically increase to high numbers around concentrated livestock operations such as dairies and calf-raising operations. Liquids such as diarrhea and milk or materials containing soluble components such as dried molasses and solid feces are attractive to nuisance flies. Because the larvae require greater than 90% humidity to develop, dampened organic calf bedding materials such as straw and sawdust provide an ideal substrate [89,90]. The ability of these insects to transmit enteric pathogens from feces is well documented [18,49]. Specific physical characteristics of flies, including mouth parts, body hairs and spines, and sticky foot pads can carry infectious agents in large numbers. Some pathogens pass through the fly digestive tract and remain viable in its feces. When feeding, the fly frequently moistens surfaces by regurgitating a "vomit drop" from its crop that contains residue, including infectious agents, from its previous meal. "Fly spots" are either such vomit drops or feces, both of which contain high numbers of infectious agents. Studies have determined that flies are attracted to diarrheic feces, that they can transmit *Cryptosporidia* in numbers higher than the minimal infectious dose for healthy humans, and that they can harbor this agent for 3 weeks after exposure [34]. Methods for controlling fly populations at different points in their life cycle have been reviewed [99]; however, it is important to point out that control methods based on chemical means alone are usually inadequate because flies readily develop resistance to such chemicals.

Rodents are also a frequently overlooked source of enteric pathogens in the farm environment. They have been implicated in the transmission of salmonellosis in dairy [98] and beef herds [44] and even in poultry flocks [20,41]. Because the feces from infected mice typically contain up to 1×10^4 salmonella per pellet [20], a single pellet may exceed the infectious dose for a susceptible calf. Current work suggests that rodents are a significant non-livestock reservoir of *Cryptosporidium*, because approximately one third of rodents of any age, even in nonlivestock ecosystems, shed *C. parvum* at an average of 1×10^3 oocysts per fecal pellet [77,101]. Importantly, significant rodent populations can be present long before their signs (e.g., rodent droppings and runways) are obvious or noticeable. Raccoons have also been reported to harbor *S.* Typhimurium [64].

Approach to minimizing risk factors related to gastrointestinal pathogens

A rational approach to management of neonatal gastrointestinal diseases of calves was first conveyed by Dr. Otto Radostits years ago [79–81] and again more recently [78]. The main tenets include management strategies directed at decreasing exposure of calves to the pathogens, increasing non-specific and specific immunity of calves, and decreasing stresses on the calves. Others have recently summarized this approach as well [39,40,70]. Although this system provides an essential foundation for addressing biosecurity for neonatal gastrointestinal diseases, further refinement suggests the following four-point approach:

1. Mitigate exposure of calves to pathogens through environmental control, monitoring, and isolation.
2. Mitigate disease severity in calves through enhancement of calf health and immunity.
3. Mitigate disease severity in calves through management of stressors placed on calves.
4. Monitor disease status within the herd through appropriate record keeping and analysis.

Mitigate exposure of calves to pathogens through environmental control, monitoring, and isolation

Those calves that are known to be particularly susceptible, either because of age or other reasons, should be isolated from each other and the rest of the herd as much as possible. Once infected, particularly if infected clinically, such calves essentially act as biological amplifiers, amplifying a small but sufficient infectious dose into a much higher level of environmental contamination in their immediate surroundings and providing a high risk for transmission through direct contact. Because this increased environmental load likely exceeds the infectious dose threshold of individuals that were resistant to the prior environmental level, more individuals become infected, the infections are more severe because of the markedly higher dose, the environmental level increases even more, and an outbreak is underway. Evidence of such a cascade is provided in one study of herds in which calves that were born after the median calving date were twice as likely to develop diarrhea than those born before it [17]. Once started, such a cascade is much more difficult to stop as compared with preventing its initiation in the first place. Evidence that members of larger groups are at increased risk of diarrhea is contained in a study of Michigan dairies, which found that the incidence of calf diarrhea was approximately proportional to herd size [32]. This finding suggests that group sizes should be minimized as much as feasible, some researchers suggesting that the ideal group size is 50 [70].

All the common agents causing neonatal calf diarrhea are often present to some degree in the calves' environment. All of the agents are primarily transmitted by fecal-oral contact, so the collective strategy for minimizing exposure of calves to pathogens should be focused on decreasing exposure to fecal contamination. Realizing that every ranch or farm has its own peculiarities regarding facilities and equipment, the following comments and suggestions should be read as general statements. Specific modifications should be individually designed to fit each production system.

Regarding dairy or beef herds calving in confined areas such as barns, the following biosecurity measures should be practiced to minimize pathogen exposure.

1. Remove late-gestation cows from areas heavily contaminated with feces, such as winter feed grounds, 1 month before calving to reduce hair coat carriage of enteric infectious agents shed by carrier cattle.
2. Separate cows requiring more intensive monitoring and thus, closer confinement, such as first-calf heifers or particularly valuable stock from those that do not.
3. Avoid moving cows into calving areas until immediately before delivery, or as late as practical.
4. Ensure that calving pens are sanitized and well bedded before and between successive calvings.
5. Clean the perineum and particularly the udder of cows before delivery.
6. Harvest colostrum from clean, sanitized udders into clean containers. Refrigerate it immediately or freeze in volumes no larger than a gallon if not administered to a calf promptly. Do not pool between dams.
7. Remove dairy calves immediately after birth and raise them in separate individual pens isolated from other calves and stock until they are older than 4 weeks.
8. Remove beef cow/calf pairs to a separate nursery area after bonding has occurred (approximately 24 hours after birth).

During the liquid-feeding phase from birth until weaning, dairy calves should be housed in individual pens or hutches to avoid contact with one another, and they should be isolated from other livestock, their airspace, and their effluent. Ideally, individual housing should be designed to prevent suckling and licking behaviors as well as fecal cross-contamination, so that transmission of enteric pathogens is minimized. The specifics regarding the construction and area requirements for dairy calves have been reviewed [57]. Calves should continue to be housed individually until 7 to 10 days after weaning. This separation allows calves to lose their suckling urge, avoids the stress at weaning of changing social structure and interactions, facilitates monitoring of feed intake during the weaning transition, and allows more accurate observations of fecal characteristics and general health [63].

Biosecurity of dairy or beef herds calving at pasture is approached with the following strategy.

1. Group primigravid heifers separately from cows during at least the last trimester of gestation.
2. Use designated calving grounds and calve heifers separately from cows. Such areas should not have been used by animals since the prior

year's calving season and should have been groomed shortly after the close of the calving season. It should be well drained and situated away from bottomlands, which tend to collect contaminants, particularly in any standing water.

3. Minimize the population density of cows as much as practical and reduce group size (<50 animals). Suggested areas per cow range from 1000 to 2000 square feet [79].

4. Remove beef cow/calf pairs to a separate nursery area after bonding but within 24 hours of calving. Exercise one-way flow regarding animal movement.

5. Rotate feeding areas during the calving season to avoid fecal contamination and pathogen build-up.

Calves demonstrating signs of lethargy or diarrhea should be removed from the group as soon as possible and placed into an isolation area. Recall the iceberg principle and consider its group of cows and calves and their area "contaminated," placing subsequently calving cows and new calves into a separate clean area. Treatments should be instituted based on physical signs and, if possible, laboratory data. Diagnostic procedures such as fecal cultures, fecal flotation, and viral identification strategies can be performed. These tests are especially important when infection with *Salmonella* spp. is a major rule out for diarrhea. Identification of rotavirus and coronavirus infection and cryptosporidiosis are arguably less essential for diagnostic purposes because in most outbreaks of acute undifferentiated diarrhea, calves frequently shed one, two, or all three of the agents simultaneously. Detection of an infectious agent in a herd known through laboratory testing to be previously free of it, however, indicates that there has been a breach of herd biosecurity. Recovering calves should be quarantined away from other animals until after the shedding of pathogens has decreased to minimal levels or for at least 3 weeks. Aside from *Salmonella* spp., the neonatal enteric pathogens with the longest shedding time are rotavirus and coronavirus, which some individuals may shed intermittently for life.

Purchased animals should be placed in separate quarantine areas before mixing with existing herd animals, especially if animals are purchased from public auctions, because the likelihood that these animals have been exposed to high doses of multiple pathogens is great. Explosive outbreaks of calf scours in beef herds are often associated with the prior purchase of a dairy calf from a sale yard to replace a calf lost because of dystocia or some other reason. A quarantine period of 21 days should be adequate to allow clinical identification of animals that are incubating any infection due to these enteric agents at the time of purchase. Quarantine of older animals for a similar period is justified because of the likelihood of increased shedding of enteric pathogens during periods of stress. Diagnostic procedures such as bacterial culture, viral detection by electron microscopy, and fecal flotation for parasite eggs can also be considered. Although it is unlikely that these tests will give a significant advantage compared with clinical observation and isolation, they can determine the etiologic agents involved. Use of such tests in older animals is less beneficial, because with the exception of *Salmonella* spp., many infected older animals shed low levels of enteric viruses. Because of the potential for false-negative results, testing may lead to a false sense of security, and management practices that are more important for establishing biosecurity may not be established and maintained.

The flow of personnel and livestock flow are important components of within-herd biosecurity [39,40,70,100]. The critical first step is to establish infection control protocols, preferably with input from those who will be responsible for executing them. Routine training and monitoring of personnel to ensure that they understand infection control protocols and that they are properly executing them are critical to biosecurity success. Because some aspects of these protocols involve significant additional effort, an understanding of why the additional effort is necessary will likely result in better adherence. Personnel and equipment flow as well as livestock flow and its effluent flow should be one-way, away from the youngest, most susceptible calves toward older, more resistant animals. On farms with sufficient personnel and equipment, tasks should be divided up between those personnel who remain "clean" for such tasks as mixing and delivering liquid feed and those who are potentially contaminated by performing tasks such as picking up empty milk bottles, treating sick calves, and so on. Personnel who are potentially contaminated through working with older or sick calves and their equipment should not return to areas with susceptible calves until they have changed their outer clothes and used appropriate procedures to thoroughly disinfect their hands, boots, and equipment. Some have recommended that calves that leave young, susceptible groups, such as for hospitalization, should not return to that group for at least 3 weeks [100].

Strict control of farm visitors must be maintained because many pathogens can be carried by humans or inanimate objects such as automobiles, tractors, livestock handling equipment, or livestock feeding equipment. For both their own and the animals' health, visitors should be discouraged from coming into contact with them or their effluent. If animal contact is necessary, visiting individuals should be provided with the means to wash their hands and footwear before and after contact. Barrier clothing should also be worn to prevent cross-contamination of separate facilities.

Mitigate disease severity in calves through enhancement of calf health and immunity

Neonatal diarrhea is a multifactorial disease process. Infection alone is not sufficient to cause disease because although almost all calves are infected shortly after birth, most do not develop clinical disease. As mentioned previously, the single strongest factor influencing the risk of death caused by neonatal calf diarrhea is the passive immune status of the calf.

The concept of failure of passive transfer has largely been used to describe situations in which the neonate does not absorb adequate levels of colostral immunoglobulins. This concept is undoubtedly attributable to the fact that immunoglobulins are such a large constituent of colostrum and they have been thoroughly studied. It is clear, however, that colostrum is a complex fluid that in addition to immunoglobulins contains various immune cells, immunoactive substances such as cytokines, and nutritional elements. Consequently, the risk of a calf contracting an enteric pathogen is a complex equation in which serum immunoglobulin concentrations are an important factor, albeit a single one.

Low immunoglobulin–concentration colostrum with the resultant ingestion of an inadequate mass of immunoglobulin is the primary cause of failure of passive transfer in dairy calves. In a study of 900 first-milking colostrums from Holstein cows, only 29% contained sufficient IgG1 concentration to provide an appropriate mass of IgG in a 2-L volume [73]. It is currently recommended that dairy calves be fed 4 liters of dairy colostrum in the first 12 hours of life to obviate the risk of failure of passive transfer caused by a lack of adequate immunoglobulin mass. To ensure intake soon enough, esophageal feeders are often used to administer these volumes.

In contrast with dairy calves, failure of passive transfer in beef calves is less likely to be due to low colostral IgG1 concentration, but rather to a failure to physically ingest and subsequently absorb the colostral immunoglobulins. Beef calves should be provided with adequate shelter during and after calving to avoid environmental stresses that lessen the calves' drive to rise and nurse. Ideally, calving should be monitored to ensure adequate mothering, which is especially important with first-calf heifers. Calves that do not rise and successfully nurse their dam within 1 to 2 hours should be assisted with nursing, or alternatively, force-fed either their dam's colostrum or frozen dairy cow colostrum. If dairy cow colostrum is used, its low average immunoglobulin concentration must be mitigated by feeding 4 liters within the first 12 hours of life. The producer must be aware that such colostrum may also be contaminated with enteric and other infectious agents (e.g., *Mycobacterium avium* subsp. *paratuberculosis*).

Mitigate disease severity in calves through management of stressors placed on calves

Stress is defined as any adverse stimulus, event, or condition, either internal or external, that disturbs an animal's physical or neurogenic homeostasis. Although there are likely numerous biological consequences of stress, a well-documented response involves the rapid and immediate increase in corticotropin secretion by the anterior pituitary gland, followed by greatly increased secretion of cortisol by the adrenal gland. Some of the beneficial effects of increased cortisol secretion include mobilization of labile proteins and fats from cellular stores for cellular energy needs, as well as numerous anti-inflammatory effects that aid in the resolution of inflammation. One of the more notable consequences of increased cortisol secretion, however, involves its extensive effects leading to immune suppression. In general, cortisol-induced atrophy of lymphoid tissues throughout the body leads to a significant decrease in both cellular and humoral immunity. It is this broad-ranging immune suppression that can lead to an increased incidence and severity of disease.

Common stresses incurred by neonatal calves include dystocia, crowding, exposure to environmental extremes such as heat, cold, or wet conditions, excessive or inappropriate handling, and exposure to pathogens [48]. Even the process of a normal parturition is a stressful condition as the fetal animal undergoes transition from intrauterine to extrauterine life. Fetal plasma cortisol levels double within minutes after uncomplicated parturition but typically decrease within the first days of life. The natural increase in plasma cortisol is necessary for normal pulmonary, intestinal, and brain development; pulmonary surfactant production; and preparation of liver glycogen stores for energy needs. Calves with dystocia are likely to have temporarily increased plasma cortisol levels and other significant laboratory abnormalities, including metabolic and respiratory acidosis and hypoglycemia [13]. Current studies indicate that the increased incidence of failure of passive transfer in calves with dystocia is not caused by a failure to absorb colostral immunoglobulins, but rather is due to the severe metabolic derangements that make these calves less likely to nurse in a timely fashion [106]. Alleviation of the stress of dystocia, therefore, should be directed toward correcting metabolic derangements and ensuring appropriate colostral intake.

Exposure to environmental extremes is likely to affect calves adversely by inhibiting normal nursing behavior and producing prolonged elevations in serum cortisol levels. Both of these factors clearly have an adverse effect on the calves' immune status, so newborn calves should be placed in sheltered environments that are free from wind and moisture and extremes of heat or cold. Providing calves with dry bedding is a critical factor in preventing problems associated with cold temperatures [69]; however, these shelters must be managed appropriately to minimize the concentration of enteric pathogens within them.

Crowding and mishandling of calves should be minimized to lessen the effect of neurogenic stress. Although limited research in this area has been undertaken in calves, it is logical to assume that calves would react similarly to other mammals in such stressful situations, with resultant increased plasma cortisol levels and subsequent immune suppression. Finally, it is logical to presume that minimizing crowding will likely not only decrease the neurogenic stress of calves but also will unquestionably decrease exposure to enteric pathogens.

Monitor disease status within the herd through record keeping and analysis

With either confined or pasture calving, it is important to keep adequate records. Records are useful for determining the timing of animal movement and for identifying the epidemiologic factors associated with sick animals as well as recording what diagnostic tests were performed, when and what treatments were administered, and their results. Particularly on larger operations, complete records maintained in a computerized database are crucial for initially determining what risk factors are associated with a neonatal diarrhea problem and then for monitoring the success of interventions.

Biosecurity, as it relates to neonatal gastrointestinal disease, should be approached as a fluid concept. Adequate records markedly enhance a producer's and a veterinarian's ability to regularly evaluate and revise neonatal disease control and prevention protocols in response to changing conditions, actual risks, and new knowledge and tools for dealing with neonatal enteric disease.

Summary

Infectious diarrhea is an important cause of neonatal calf morbidity and mortality that results in significant economic losses in the beef and dairy industries. Although numerous risk factors related to the occurrence of neonatal diarrhea have been identified, they can all be categorized into those that are related to the calf, the pathogens involved, or the environment of the calf. The immune status of calves, specifically the level of passively acquired immunity through colostrum, is the major risk factor related to the calf and the occurrence of diarrhea. Although numerous pathogens have been implicated in the occurrence of neonatal diarrhea, only a relatively limited number are commonly involved. Most should be viewed as secondary opportunists rather than primary pathogens, because none are extraordinarily virulent, and with the exception of *Salmonella* spp., most are present within the gastrointestinal tract of many healthy, mature cattle. Important risk factors related to pathogens involved in neonatal calf diarrhea involve the size of the inoculum and the occurrence of multiple infections. Finally, when considering the environment and housing conditions in which beef and dairy calves may reside, it is clear that tremendous variations exist. Despite these variations, the risk factors associated with the environment of the calf are also those that are the most amenable to the implementation of general environmental control and monitoring strategies as well as specific biosecurity measures.

References

[1] Acres SD, Saunders J, Radostits OM. Acute undifferentiated neonatal diarrhea of beef calves: the prevalence of enterotoxigenic *E. coli*, reo-like (rota) virus and other enteropathogens in cow-calf herds. Can Vet J 1977;18:113–21.

[2] Anderson BC. Effect of drying on the infectivity of cryptosporidia-laden calf feces for 3- to 7-day-old mice. Am J Vet Res 1986;47:2272–3.

[3] Anderson BC. Moist heat inactivation of *Cryptosporidium* sp. Am J Public Health 1985;75:1433–4.

[4] Anderson JF. Biosecurity—a new term for an old concept: how to apply it. The Bovine Practitioner 1998;32:61–70.

[5] Anderson JF, Bates DW. Influence of improved ventilation on health of confined cattle. J Am Vet Med Assoc 1979;174:577–80.

[6] Atwill ER, Harp JA, Jones T, Jardon PW, Checel S, Zylstra M. Evaluation of peri- parturient dairy cows and contact surfaces as a reservoir of *Cryptosporidium parvum* for calfhood infection. Am J Vet Res 1998;59:1116–21.

[7] Atwill ER, Johnson EM, Pereira MG. Association of herd composition, stocking rate, and duration of calving season with fecal shedding of *Cryptosporidium parvum* oocysts in beef herds. J Am Vet Med Assoc 1999;215:1833–8.

[8] Bale MJ, Bennett PM, Beringer JE, Hinton M. The survival of bacteria exposed to desiccation on surfaces associated with farm buildings. J Appl Bacteriol 1993;75:519–28.

[9] Bates DW, Anderson JF. Calculation of ventilation needs for confined cattle. J Am Vet Med Assoc 1979;174:581–9.

[10] Beef Cow/Calf Health and Productivity Audit. Part III. Beef Cow/Calf Health and Health Management, January 1994. Fort Collins (CO): US Department of Agriculture, Animal and Plant Inspection Service, Veterinary Services, National Animal Health Monitoring System; 1994. p. 37.

[11] Bendali F, Sanaa M, Bichet H, Schelcher F. Risk factors associated with diarrhoea in newborn calves. Vet Res 1999;30:509–22.

[12] Besser TE, Gay CC. The importance of colostrum to the health of the neonatal calf. Vet Clin North Am Food Anim Pract 1994;10:107–17.

[13] Breazile JE, Vollmer LA, Rice LE. Neonatal adaptation to stress of parturition and dystocia. Vet Clin North Am Food Anim Pract 1988;4:481–99.

[14] Campbell I, Tzipori AS, Hutchison G, Angus KW. Effect of disinfectants on survival of cryptosporidium oocysts. Vet Rec 1982;111:414–5.

[15] Chauret C, Nolan K, Chen P, Springthorpe S, Sattar S. Aging of *Cryptosporidium parvum* oocysts in river water and their susceptibility to disinfection by chlorine and mono- chloramine. Can J Microbiol 1998;44:1154–60.

[16] Cho KO, Halbur PG, Bruna JD, Sorden SD, Yoon KJ, Janke BH, et al. Detection and isolation of coronavirus from feces of three herds of feedlot cattle during outbreaks of winter dysentery-like disease. J Am Vet Med Assoc 2000;217:1191–4.

[17] Clement JC, King ME, Salman MD, Wittum TE, Casper HH, Odde KG. Use of epidemiologic principles to identify risk factors associated with the development of diarrhea in calves in five beef herds. J Am Vet Med Assoc 1995;207:1334–8.

[18] Cohen D, Green M, Block C, Slepan R, Ambar R, Wasserman SS, et al. Reduction of transmission of shigellosis by control of houseflies (*Musca domestica*). Lancet 1991; 337:993–7.

[19] Crouch CF, Oliver S, Hearle DC, Buckley A, Chapman AJ, Francis MJ. Lactogenic im- munity following vaccination of cattle with bovine coronavirus. Vaccine 2000;19:189–96.

[20] Davies RH, Wray C. Mice as carriers of *Salmonella enteritidis* on persistently infected poultry units. Vet Rec 1995;137:337–41.

[21] Davis CL, Drackley JK. The development, nutrition and management of the young calf. Ames (IA): Iowa State University Press; 1998.

[22] de Graaf DC, Vanopdenbosch E, Ortega-Mora LM, Abbassi H, Peeters JE. A review of the importance of cryptosporidiosis in farm animals. Int J Parasitol 1999;29: 1269–87.

[23] Dennehy PH. Transmission of rotavirus and other enteric pathogens in the home. Pediatr Infect Dis J 2000;19(10 Suppl):S103–S105.

[24] Donaldson AI. Factors influencing the dispersal, survival and deposition of airborne pathogens of farm animals. Vet Bull 1978;48:83–94.

[25] Donovan GA. Evaluation of dairy heifer replacement-rearing programs. Compend Cont Ed Pract Vet 1987;9:F133–F139.

[26] Evans S, Davies R. Case control study of multiple-resistant *Salmonella typhimurium* DT104 infection of cattle in Great Britain. Vet Rec 1996;139:557–8.

[27] Evermann JF, Benfield DA. Coronaviral infections. In: Williams ES, Barber IK, editors. Infectious diseases of wild mammals, 3rd edition. Ames (IA): Iowa State University Press; 2001. p. 245–53.

[28] Evermann JF. Pregnancy-associated immunodeficiency. In: Smith BP, editor. Large animal internal medicine, 3rd edition. St. Louis: Mosby; 2002. p. 1603–4.

[29] Fayer R, Morgan U, Upton SJ. Epidemiology of *Cryptosporidium*: transmission, detection and identification. Int J Parasitol 2000;30:1305–22.

[30] Fayer R, Nerad T. Effects of low temperatures on viability of *Cryptosporidium parvum* oocysts. Appl Environ Microbiol 1996;62:1431–3.

[31] Foster JW, Spector MP. How Salmonella survive against the odds. Annu Rev Microbiol 1995;49:145–74.

[32] Frank NA, Kaneene JB. Management risk factors associated with calf diarrhea in Michigan dairy herds. J Dairy Sci 1993;76:1313–23.

[33] Garcia A, Ruiz-Santa-Quiteria JA, Orden JA, Cid D, Sanz R, Gomez-Bautista M, et al. Rotavirus and concurrent infections with other enteropathogens in neonatal diarrheic dairy calves in Spain. Comp Immunol Microbiol Infect Dis 2000;23:175–83.

[34] Graczyk TK, Fayer R, Knight R, Mhangami-Ruwende B, Trout JM, Da Silva AJ, et al. Mechanical transport and transmission of *Cryptosporidium parvum* oocysts by wild filth flies. Am J Trop Med Hyg 2000;63:178–83.

[35] Graczyk TK, Knight R, Gilman RH, Cranfield MR. The role of non-biting flies in the epidemiology of human infectious diseases. Microbes Infect 2001;3:231–5.

[36] Graham DY, Dufour GR, Estes MK. Minimal infective dose of rotavirus. Arch Virol 1987;92:261–71.

[37] Hand MS, Hunt E, Phillips RW. Milk replacers for the neonatal calf. Vet Clin North Am Food Anim Pract 1985;1:589–608.

[38] Hardman PM, Wathes CM, Wray C. Transmission of Salmonellae among calves penned individually. Vet Rec 1991;129:327–9.

[39] Heath SE. Neonatal diarrhea in calves: investigation of herd management practices. Cont Ed Pract Vet 1992;14:385–393.

[40] Heath SE. Neonatal diarrhea in calves: diagnosis and intervention in problem herds. Cont Ed Pract Vet 1992;14:995–1002.

[41] Henzler DJ, Opitz HM. The role of mice in the epizootiology of *Salmonella enteritidis* infection on chicken layer farms. Avian Dis 1992;36:625–31.

[42] Himathongkham S, Bahari S, Riemann H, Cliver D. Survival of *Escherichia coli* O157:H7 and *Salmonella typhimurium* in cow manure and cow manure slurry. FEMS Microbiol Lett 1999;178:251–7.

[43] Hunt E. Foreword. Vet Clin North Am Food Anim Pract 1985;1:443.

[44] Hunter AG, Linklater KA, Scott JA. Rodent vectors of Salmonella. Vet Rec 1976;99:145–6.

[45] Jamaluddin AA, Hird DW, Thurmond MC, Carpenter TE. Effect of preweaning feeding of pasteurized and nonpasteurized milk on postweaning weight gain of heifer calves on a Californian dairy. Prev Vet Med 1996;28:91–9.

[46] Kahrs RF. General disinfection guidelines. Rev Sci Tech 1995;14:105–63.

[47] Kahrs RF. Rotavirus associated with neonatal diarrhea. In: Kahrs RF, editor. Viral diseases of cattle, 2nd edition. Ames (IA): Iowa State University Press; 2001. p. 239–46.

[48] Kasari TR, Wikse SE. Perinatal mortality in beef herds. Vet Clin North Am Food Anim Pract 1994;10:1–180.

[49] Kettle DS. Introduction. In: Medical and veterinary entomology, 2nd edition. Wallingford, Oxon, UK: CAB International; 1995. p. 3–12.

[50] Larson EL. APIC guideline for handwashing and hand antisepsis in health care settings. Am J Infect Control 1995;23:251–69.

[51] Lederberg J. Emerging infections: an evolutionary perspective. Emerg Infect Dis 1998;4: 366–71.

[52] Lederberg J. Infectious disease as an evolutionary paradigm. Emerg Infect Dis 1997;3: 417–23.

[53] Levine MM. *Escherichia coli* that cause diarrhea: enterotoxigenic, enteropathogenic, enteroinvasive, enterohemorrhagic and enteroadherent. J Infect Dis 1987;155:377–89.

[54] Linton AH, Hugo WB, Russell AD. Chemical disinfectants. In: Disinfection in veterinary and farm animal practice. Oxford: Blackwell Scientific; 1987. p. 12–42.

[55] Lorenzo MJ, Ares-Mazas E, Villacorta Martinez de Maturana I. Detection of oocysts and IgG antibodies to *Cryptosporidium parvum* in asymptomatic adult cattle. Vet Parasitol 1993;47:9–15.

[56] McDonough SP, Stull CL, Osburn BI. Enteric pathogens in intensively reared veal calves. Am J Vet Res 1994;55:1516–20.

[57] McFarland DF. Housing calves: birth to weaning. In: Calves, heifers and dairy profitability: facilities, nutrition and health. publication no. 74. Ithaca (NY): Northeast Regional Agricultural Engineering Service; 1996. p. 82–9.

[58] Mitscherlich E, Marth EH. *E. coli*. In: Microbial survival in the environment. New York: Springer-Verlag; 1984. p. 166–84.

[59] Moe K, Shirley JA. The effects of relative humidity and temperature on the survival of human rotavirus in faeces. Arch Virol 1982;72:179–86.

[60] Mohammed HO, Wade SE, Schaaf S. Risk factors associated with *Cryptosporidium parvum* infection in dairy cattle in southeastern New York State. Vet Parasitol 1999;83:1–13.

[61] Moon HW, McClurkin AW, Isaacson RE, Pohlenz J, Skartvedt SM, Gillette KG, et al. Pathogenic relationships of rotavirus, *Escherichia coli*, and other agents in mixed infections in calves. J Am Vet Med Assoc 1978;173:577–83.

[62] Morgan-Jones SC. Cleansing and disinfection of farm buildings. In: Collins CH, Allwood MC, Bloomfield SF, Fox A, editors. Disinfectants: their use and evaluation of effectiveness New York: Academic Press; 1981. p. 199–212.

[63] Morrill JL. The calf: birth to 12 weeks. In: Van Horn HH, Wilcox CJ, editors. Large dairy herd management. Champaign (IL): American Dairy Science Association; 1992. p. 401–10.

[64] Morse EV, Midla DA, Kazacos KR. Raccoons (*Procyon lotor*) as carriers of Salmonella. J Environ Sci Health A 1983;18:541–60.

[65] National Dairy Heifer Evaluation Project. Dairy heifer morbidity, mortality, and health management focusing on preweaned heifers, April 1991–July 1992. Fort Collins (CO): US Department of Agriculture, Animal Plant Inspection Service, Veterinary Services, National Animal Health Monitoring Service; 1994. p. 4–10.

[66] Naylor JM. Neonatal ruminant diarrhea. In: Smith BP, editor. Large animal internal medicine, 2nd edition. St. Louis: Mosby; 1996. p. 396–417.

[67] Olson DP, Bull RC, Kelly KW, Riter RC, Woodard LF, Everson DO. Effects of maternal nutrition restriction and cold stress on young calves: Clinical condition, behavioral reactions, and lesions. Am J Vet Res 1981;42:758–63.

[68] O'Mahony J, O'Donoghue M, Morgan JG, Hill C. Rotavirus survival and stability in foods as determined by an optimised plaque assay procedure. Int J Food Microbiol 2000;61:177–85.

[69] Pelton JA, Barrington GM, Callan RJ, Parish SM. Frostbite in calves. Comp Cont Ed Pract Vet 2000;22:S136–S141.

[70] Pence M, Robbe S, Thomson J. Reducing the incidence of neonatal calf diarrhea through evidence-based management. Comp Cont Ed Pract Vet 2001;23:S73–S75.

[71] Perino LJ. A guide to colostrum management in beef cows and calves. Vet Med 1997; 92:75–82.

[72] Plym-Forshell L, Ekesbo I. Survival of salmonellas in urine and dry faeces from cattle: An experimental study. Acta Vet Scand 1996;37:127–31.

[73] Pritchett LC, Gay CC, Besser TE, Hancock DD. Management and production factors influencing immunoglobulin G1 concentration in colostrum from Holstein cows. J Dairy Sci 1991;74:2336–41.

[74] Prokop A, Humphrey AE. Kinetics of disinfection. In: Benarde ME, editor. Disinfection. New York: Marcel Dekker; 1970. p. 61–8.

[75] Quigley JD, Drewry JJ. Nutrient and immunity transfer from cow to calf pre- and postcalving. J Dairy Sci 1998;81:2779–90.

[76] Quigley JD, Martin KR, Bemis DA, Potgieter LN, Reinemeyer CR, Rohrbach BW, et al. Effects of housing and colostrum feeding on the prevalence of selected infectious organisms in feces of Jersey calves. J Dairy Sci 1994;77:3124–31.

[77] Quy RJ, Cowan DP, Haynes PJ, Sturdee AP, Chalmers RM, Bodely-Tickell AT, et al. The Norway rat as a reservoir host of *Cryptosporidium parvum.* J Wildl Dis 1999;35: 660–70.

[78] Radostits OM, editor. Herd health: food animal production medicine, 3rd edition. Philadelphia: WB Saunders; 2001. p. 333–95.

[79] Radostits OM. The role of management and the use of vaccines in the control of acute undifferentiated diarrhea of newborn calves. Can Vet J 1991;32:155–9.

[80] Radostits OM, Acres SD. The control of acute undifferentiated diarrhea of newborn beef calves. Vet Clin North Am Large Anim Pract 1983;5:143–55.

[81] Radostits OM, Acres SD. The prevention and control of epidemics of acute undifferentiated diarrhea of beef calves in western Canada. Can Vet J 1980;21:243–9.

[82] Radostits OM, Bell JM. Nutrition of the pre-ruminant dairy calf with special reference to the digestion and absorption of nutrients: A review. Can J Anim Sci 1970;50: 405–52.

[83] Radostits OM, Blood DC. Nutrition. In: Herd health: a textbook of health and production management of agricultural animals. Philadelphia: WB Saunders; 1985. p. 134–73.

[84] Raphael RA, Sattar SA, Springthorpe VS. Long-term survival of human rotavirus in raw and treated river water. Can J Microbiol 1985;31:124–8.

[85] Reynolds DJ, Morgan JH, Chanter N, Jones PW, Bridger JC, Debney TG, et al. Microbiology of calf diarrhoea in southern Britain. Vet Rec 1986;119:34–9.

[86] Robertson LJ, Campbell AT, Smith HV. Survival of *Cryptosporidium parvum* oocysts under various environmental pressures. Appl Environ Microbiol 1992;58:3494–500.

[87] Rutala WA, Weber DJ. Uses of inorganic hypochlorite (bleach) in health-care facilities. Clin Microbiol Rev 1997;10:597–610.

[88] Sanderson MW, Dargatz DA. Risk factors for high herd level calf morbidity risk from birth to weaning in beef herds in the USA. Prev Vet Med 2000;44:97–106.

[89] Schmidtmann ET. Exploitation of bedding in dairy outdoor calf hutches by immature house and stable flies (Diptera: Muscidae). J Med Entomol 1988;25:484–8.

[90] Schmidtmann ET. Suppressing immature house and stable flies in outdoor calf hutches with sand, gravel, and sawdust bedding. J Dairy Sci 1991;74:3956–60.

[91] Schumann FJ, Townsend HG, Naylor JM. Risk factors for mortality from diarrhea in beef calves in Alberta. Can J Vet Res 1990;54:366–72.

[92] Scott CA, Smith HV, Mtambo MM, Gibbs HA. An epidemiological study of *Cryptosporidium parvum* in two herds of adult beef cattle. Vet Parasitol 1995;57:277–88.

[93] Scott FW. Virucidal disinfectants and feline viruses. Am J Vet Res 1980;41:410–4.

[94] Selim SA, Cullor JS. Number of viable bacteria and presumptive antibiotic residues in milk fed to calves on commercial dairies. J Am Vet Med Assoc 1997;211:1029–35.

[95] Sivula NJ, Ames TR, Marsh WE. Management practices and risk factors for morbidity and mortality in Minnesota dairy heifer calves. Prev Vet Med 1996;27:173–82.

[96] Snodgrass DR, Terzolo HR, Sherwood D, Campbell I, Menzies JD, Synge BA. Aetiology of diarrhea in young calves. Vet Rec 1986;119:31–4.

[97] Storz J, Lin X, Purdy CW, Chouljenko VN, Kousoulas KG, Enright FM, et al. Coronavirus and *Pasteurella* infections in bovine shipping fever pneumonia and Evans' criteria for causation. J Clin Microbiol 2000;38:3291–8.

[98] Tablante NL, Lane VM. Wild mice as potential reservoirs of *Salmonella dublin* in a closed dairy herd. Can Vet J 1989;30:590–2.

[99] Thomas G, Jespersen JB. Non-biting Muscidae and control methods. Rev Sci Tech 1994;13:1159–73.

[100] Thomson JU. Implementing biosecurity in beef and dairy operations. Proceedings of the Thirtieth Annual Conference American Association of Bovine Practitioners 1997;30: 8–14.

[101] Torres J, Gracenea M, Gomez MS, Arrizabalaga A, Gonzalez-Moreno O. The occurrence of *Cryptosporidium parvum* and *C. muris* in wild rodents and insectivores in Spain. Vet Parasitol 2000;92:253–60.

[102] Waltner-Toews D, Martin SW, Meek AH. An epidemiological study of selected calf pathogens on Holstein dairy farms in southwestern Ontario. Can Vet J 1986;50:307–13.

[103] Ward RL, Bernstein DI, Young EC, Sherwood JR, Knowlton DR, Schiff GM. Human rotavirus studies in volunteers: determination of infectious dose and serological response to infection. J Infect Dis 1986;154:871–80.

[104] Wathes CM, Jones CD, Webster AJ. Ventilation, air hygiene and animal health. Vet Rec 1983;113:554–9.

[105] Wathes CM, Zaidan WA, Pearson GR, Hinton M, Todd N. Aerosol infection of calves and mice with *Salmonella typhimurium*. Vet Rec 1988;123:590–4.

[106] Weaver DM, Tyler JW, VanMetre DC, Hostetler DE, Barrington GM. Passive transfer of colostral immunoglobulins in calves. J Vet Intern Med 2000;14:569–77.

[107] Weber DJ, Rutala WA. The emerging nosocomial pathogens *Cryptosporidium*, *Escherichia coli* O157:H7, *Helicobacter pylori*, and hepatitis C: epidemiology, environmental survival, efficacy of disinfection, and control measures. Infect Control Hosp Epidemiol 2001;22:306–15.

[108] Wells SJ, Dargatz DA, Ott SL. Factors associated with mortality to 21 days of life in dairy heifers in the United States. Prev Vet Med 1996;29:9–19.

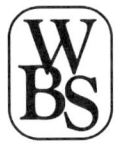

Vet Clin Food Anim 18 (2002) 35–55

THE VETERINARY
CLINICS
Food Animal
Practice

Biosecurity for gastrointestinal diseases of adult dairy cattle

Scott J. Wells, DVM, PhD*, Scott Dee, DVM, PhD,
Sandra Godden, BSC, DVM, DVsc

*Department of Clinical and Population Sciences, University of Minnesota,
College of Veterinary Medicine, 1365 Gortner Avenue, St. Paul, MN 55108, USA*

Perhaps no one single factor has the ability to affect the performance of animal populations as severely as infectious disease. Exposure to bacterial and viral pathogens occurs frequently in the life of an individual animal and can spread laterally throughout large populations at a rapid rate. Depending on the level of immunity within the population and the degree of management under which the animals are raised, the effect can be quite severe, particularly if concurrent infection of multiple pathogens should occur. The need to prevent the introduction of and to mitigate the effects of such pathogens has resulted in the evolution of disease-control strategies and biosecurity programs. It is a misconception that only large production units can afford to take advantage of advanced principles of disease control. The practice of biosecurity and the application of disease detection techniques are important to all producers.

The preceding paragraph is entirely appropriate for cattle herds, but it is also applicable (and was originally written) for swine farms. As biosecurity management strategies are developed and implemented to prevent introduction and spread of infectious diseases in cattle populations, it is informative to review principles of biosecurity from another livestock species in which these issues have been considered (e.g., swine) and compare these perspectives to the current situation for cattle. Should cattle biosecurity programs of the future adapt parts of the swine biosecurity model? To address this question, the authors follow a biosecurity risk-assessment model to identify important health hazards, evaluate risks, and present principles for implementing a cattle biosecurity program for important gastrointestinal health hazards of adult dairy cattle, after consideration of a swine biosecurity model.

---

* Corresponding author.
E-mail address: wells023@tc.umn.edu (S.J. Wells).

0749-0720/02/$ - see front matter © 2002, Elsevier Science (USA). All rights reserved.
PII: S 0 7 4 9 - 0 7 2 0 (0 2) 0 0 0 0 7 - 5

Use of a risk-assessment approach to evaluate biosecurity risks for cattle populations

Biosecurity can be defined as a strategy to control and prevent animal and public health-related losses. Development of a biosecurity management plan on dairy operations using a risk-assessment process has been described previously [26], categorizing the microbial risk assessment process into components of hazard identification, exposure assessment, dose-response assessment, and risk characterization [3]. Available information dictates the validity and precision of the risk estimates generated.

Hazard identification

A prioritization process for important diseases and health conditions of dairy cattle has recently been described [29], considering hazards with associated production losses, zoonotic potential, international trade implications, and animal welfare concerns. A similar process should be evaluated from the individual perspective of each cattle operation, considering the most important hazards to sustainable profitability of the enterprise. Primary pathogens of concern may differ from herd to herd, depending on factors such as sale of breeding stock. For many dairy cattle producers, the adult cow gastrointestinal pathogens of highest concern include *Mycobacterium paratuberculosis* (*M. avium* subsp. *paratuberculosis*, the cause of Johne's disease) and *Salmonella* spp. These pathogens therefore form the basis for much of the biosecurity discussion that follows.

Johne's disease and salmonellosis are of increasing concern as cattle become more concentrated within herds of large cow numbers. Animal movements from farm to farm, especially herd expansions, create special pathogen risks owing to increased exposures of cattle to multiple pathogens at times of reduced immune function related to stresses of transportation and animal re-sorting. Also, dairy cattle in the United States have become more genetically homogeneous [10], leading to risks of lack of hybrid vigor and associated lack of resistance to diseases to which these cattle are exposed. The authors begin by evaluating the disease effect, epidemiology (reservoirs of infection, primary methods of transmission), and primary control measures of these two cattle diseases. More complete understanding of the epidemiology of disease can lead to the development and implementation of more effective control strategies through the interruption of transmission between and within farms.

Economic losses from Johne's disease primarily are related to impaired animal health in affected herds (reduced milk production and premature involuntary culling in affected cattle, with resulting losses of over $200 per cow in heavily infected herds) [16] but also may include loss of livestock sales due to buyer concerns about the disease and potential future concerns about uncertain public health risks. Cattle serve as a primary reservoir of infection for *M. paratuberculosis*, the pathogen causing Johne's disease, along with other ruminant species and potentially, other animals. *M. paratuberculosis* is an intracellular bacterium that survives well but does not replicate outside infected animals for extended periods [5]. Transmission to uninfected cattle occurs primarily through fecal-oral routes and also through consumption of contaminated or infected milk, colostrum, or water [22]. Young calves are at highest risk of becoming infected. A long incubation period of 3 to 6 years precedes development of clinical signs. Factors predisposing to transmission of Johne's disease include introduction of cattle to the herd and use of management practices that expose young replacement heifers to the pathogen (use of multiple-cow maternity areas, lack of segregation of calves from dams after birth, and feeding of contaminated colostrum and milk to calves) [8,27]. Because of the epidemiology of Johne's disease (highest susceptibility of youngest cattle and long incubation period before clinical disease), reduction of exposure of youngstock to the pathogen is of primary importance in dairy herd control programs.

Economic losses from *Salmonella* spp. occur because of clinical disease and mortality in cattle of all ages, but an even larger potential effect is the growing public health concern about *Salmonella* spp. as a critical and costly food-borne pathogen of humans. Recently, concern has arisen from the public health community about the emergence of antibiotic-resistant strains of *Salmonella* spp. One of these strains (*Salmonella* Typhimurium DT104) was recognized in the 1990s in the United States and elsewhere as characteristically resistant to five different antimicrobics and associated with disease outbreaks in humans and cattle [1]. Salmonellosis is caused by the bacterium *Salmonella enterica*, with more than 2200 serotypes identified. The reservoir of infection includes all species of animals and birds [17]. These pathogens also can replicate in the environment under certain temperature and moisture conditions out of direct sunlight and can survive for several months [14,18]. Transmission occurs primarily through fecal-oral routes, often through contaminated feed, water, or the environment. The epidemiology of *Salmonella* spp. transmission can be complex, however, with transmission cycling though multiple species of animals in a geographic area, as demonstrated by Kinde et al. [12]. Risk factors for dairy cattle include introduction of infected cattle, grouping and housing of cattle, contaminated feed and water, and transfer of the pathogen by movement of vehicles, people, rodents, birds, and other animals [18,25]. Control of *Salmonella* spp. transmission is especially challenging because the organism can persist in cattle environments [7].

All cattle producers should consider prevention of unusual disease outbreaks, including those diseases classified as foreign to their country. Foreign animal diseases with gastrointestinal clinical signs include such diseases as rinderpest, which is internationally reportable as an Office International des Epizooties List A disease based on the potential for serious socioeconomic or public health consequences. The risk of rinderpest due to movement of cattle is low in North America because of the geographic isolation of North America from much of the rest of the world, strict regulation of animal movements from infected countries, and lack of carrier state in recovered cattle [24]. Other foreign animal diseases, however, pose higher risks of transmission through the international movement of animals, people, animal products, or semen and embryos.

Exposure assessment

Risk of exposure to pathogens is related to prevalence of the pathogens in various cattle populations and the probability of exposure to those cattle populations. Both Johne's disease and salmonellosis are endemic to North America and commonly identified in dairy herds. The National Animal Health Monitoring System (NAHMS) has estimated that at least 22% of US dairy herds and 8% of US beef cow–calf herds are infected with *M. paratuberculosis* [6,27]. Cow-level estimates of infection are conservative because of a lack of sensitivity of current diagnostic tests early in the course of infection, but the NAHMS estimates that 2% to 4% of US dairy cattle are infected as well as 0.4% of US beef cattle [4].

From the 1996 NAHMS Dairy Study [28], milk cows on 21% of dairies were shedding *Salmonella* spp. in feces at detectable levels using fecal culture at a single visit, including 5% of milk cows. From this study, in herds with at least 100 milk cows, nearly 9% of cows were shedding *Salmonella* spp. at detectable levels compared with 0.6% of cows from herds with less than 100 milk cows. These estimates are expected to be conservative estimates of the true prevalence of infection, because cows on 75% of large California dairies have been shown to have serologic evidence of exposure to *Salmonella* [21].

From recent NAHMS national studies, estimates of use of certain biosecurity practices for dairy and beef cattle can be obtained. A summarization of some practices used in the US dairy cattle population (Table 1) clearly indicates the potential risk of disease introduction through widespread lapses in between-herd biosecurity. Depending on herd size, 41% to 66% of US dairy operations introduce cattle to their operations each year, with little use of isolation or quarantine before introduction and little testing for exposure to certain pathogens before introduction. Isolation of incoming cattle before introduction to the herd is not an effective control measure for diseases of long incubation like Johne's disease, but it can be effective for diseases with shorter incubation periods, including salmonellosis. Although many cattle producers identify animals for herd management purposes, no universal animal identification exists to track the movement of cattle from farm to farm. Such systems have been adopted in Canada and parts of Europe, and tracking movements could facilitate control of certain diseases.

Likewise, risks of pathogen spread from older to younger naive cattle within a herd are generally high in US dairy herds (Table 2). Use of multiple-cow maternity housing systems is common and presents an ideal mechanism for transmission of infection with *M. paratuberculosis* and *Salmonella* spp. (and many other pathogens) from cows to susceptible calves.

Table 1
Use of between-herd management practices related to between-herd control of infectious disease by herd size

Management practices	Operations (%)		
	No. of milking cows		
	<100	100–200	>200
Introduce the following cattle onto the operation in previous year			
Bred dairy heifers	15	26	48
Lactating dairy cows	19	23	26
Bulls (weaned)	7	13	23
Any dairy or beef cattle	41	52	66
Operation average percent of cow inventory brought on the operation in the previous year (of operations that brought cattle onto the operation)			
Cows	19	16	12
Heifers	17	13	20
No quarantine of cattle for at least 7 days (of operations that brought the following cattle onto the operation in previous year)			
Bred dairy heifers	89	87	82
Lactating dairy cows	96	99	89
Bulls (weaned)	89	93	88
Not normally required before bringing cattle on farm (of operations that brought cattle onto the operation in previous year)			
M. paratuberculosis test	91	85	95
BVD virus test	85	78	86
BVD virus vaccination	57	41	41
Cattle left the operation for fairs and shows and returned to the operation in previous year	16	24	26

From Wells SJ. Biosecurity on dairy operations: hazards and risks. J Dairy Sci 2000;83:1–7; with permission.

Maternity pens are often used as housing for sick and lame cattle, increasing risks of calf exposure. Equipment is sometimes used for cattle feed and manure handling, potentially contaminating feed before consumption, and some operations use recycled water to flush cow alleyways, both practices potentially perpetuating the cycle of fecal-oral pathogens in cattle environments.

US dairy herds are currently managed in a manner that presents multiple opportunities for introduction of pathogens, including *M. paratuberculosis* and *Salmonella* spp. A few of these risks have been estimated previously. Introduction of 40 cows to a dairy herd from herds of unknown Johne's disease health status leads to a 65% probability of introducing Johne's disease

Table 2
Use of management practices related to within-herd control of infectious disease by herd size

| | Operations (%) | | |
| | No. of milking cows | | |
Management Practice	<100	100–200	>200
Use of multiple-cow maternity housing facilities	47	63	72
Use of maternity housing not separate from that of lactating dairy cows	61	31	13
Frequent or occasional use of calving area as a hospital area for sick cows	56	58	43
At least 25% of heifer calves born on the operation remained with their dams more than 24 hours	17	11	10
Use of multiple-calf preweaned heifer housing	50	31	33
Equipment used for manure handling also used to handle feed given to heifers <12 months of age			
At least weekly	11	19	13
Occasionally but less than weekly	10	12	14
Sick cows not separated from other cows and heifers to prevent nose-to-nose contact	86	76	53

From Wells SJ. Biosecurity on dairy operations: hazards and risks. J Dairy Sci 2000;83:1–7; with permission.

to the herd [26]. Use of flush systems for cow alleyways is associated with a 33% to 90% probability of herd infection with *Salmonella*, depending on ration and herd location [11].

Dose-response assessment

Limited information suggests that dose of pathogen plays a role in development of Johne's disease and salmonellosis. Young cattle develop more extensive lesions after experimental exposure to *M. paratuberculosis* than older cattle [13], indicating the effect of timing of exposure to *M. paratuberculosis* on infectious dose. Clinically ill cattle may shed more than 10^8 bacilli per gram of feces and up to 5×10^{12} bacilli per day [5], indicating the massive dose potentially received. The infectious dose of *Salmonella* spp. likely is dependent on serotype, virulence of strain, and the age of cattle host [17]. A single cow may shed 10^6 *S.* Dublin organisms per gram of feces and 10^9 organisms per day [18].

Risk characterization

Although quantitative risk estimates are not available for these diseases, the morbidity and mortality caused by Johne's disease and salmonellosis indicate the relative ease of transmission. A qualitative approach to evaluate the risk of transmission has been developed for Johne's disease as outlined in the following section.

Risk-assessment approach for Johne's disease

It is important for each producer who chooses to focus on Johne's disease to evaluate the most important transmission risks within the herd and then develop a herd plan to deal with highest risk management areas. The format for a Johne's disease risk assessment was initially developed and endorsed by the National Johne's Working Group and more recently modified in Minnesota to create a working system for use on-farm by veterinarians (www.cvm.umn.edu/dairycenter/johnes). This risk assessment, continuing to be developed to improve standardization, provides a useful method of assessing the priority areas of risk of transmission to various cattle age groups with *M. paratuberculosis*. The risk assessment is weighted to focus attention on the maternity pen and young replacement heifers (such as early separation of calf from dam) because of the biology of Johne's disease. Adoption of a herd biosecurity plan to address the highest risk areas should also prevent transmission of many other diseases such as salmonellosis and rotaviral and coronaviral infections.

To expand the herd plan from Johne's disease to prevention of *Salmonella* spp infections, it is important to expand the biosecurity focus to other areas as well, although retaining the focus on exposure by cattle to fecal material. Smith and House [20] have proposed priority areas for focus in reduction of *Salmonella* transmission using a best management practice approach. Although model *Salmonella* control programs in dairy herds have not yet been demonstrated to be effective in practice, the authors expect that successful pathogen reduction programs of the future will include many of the areas emphasized by Smith and House.

Risk management: applying biosecurity principles for cattle populations

Putting these ideas into action is the risk management part of the equation. Using the outline developed in our swine biosecurity model (found in the Appendix at the end of this article), the authors consider a strategy designed to reduce the risk of pathogen introduction to and within farms in the development of a comprehensive framework of biosecurity directed especially toward the pathogens *M. paratuberculosis* and *Salmonella* spp. in dairy cattle herds.

Health status of the dairy herd

Veterinarians should work with the herd management team to develop protocols for the routine monitoring, diagnosis, and treatment of common diseases. Development of protocols in this manner ensures that planning takes place with input from all of the important players and also ensures that this plan is communicated to everyone involved. Although these services and programs are more likely to be requested by mid- and large-sized dairies, smaller dairies also can use them successfully. For Johne's disease and salmonellosis, the first level of monitoring is the recording of clinical cases of disease. Most cows with clinical Johne's disease (diarrhea and weight loss not responsive to treatment) are culled from the herd, so a record of clinical Johne's disease as a contributing cause for culling is an efficient way to measure the incidence of Johne's disease in the herd through time. Similarly, for salmonellosis, occurrence of acute cases of enteritis and mortality in calves and older cattle should be recorded and followed up with diagnostic evaluations to determine etiology.

Routine diagnostic evaluations of clinically abnormal animals are recommended, either by the herd veterinarian or by trained and skilled herd managers using diagnostic protocols developed with the herd veterinarian. All dead animals, including youngstock and adults, should be routinely necropsied by the herd veterinarian, and appropriate samples should be submitted to the regional veterinary diagnostic laboratory. Record-keeping systems, whether paper or electronic in nature, should be in place, with all cases of morbidity and mortality routinely recorded. The management team, including the herd veterinarian, should review records of production and disease on a regular basis. Only by having such monitoring and record-keeping programs in place will producers be able to detect early occurrences of unusual disease incursions in the herd.

Monitoring of infection and exposure to Johne's disease and *Salmonella* is helpful in developing and evaluating progress with the biosecurity plan. For Johne's disease, the initial step is to confirm the presence or absence of *M. paratuberculosis* on the operation. ELISA tests can be used as herd screening tests, but they need to be followed up with fecal culture to confirm infection in the herd. Lack of confirmed infection with *M. paratuberculosis* leads biosecurity planning in a different direction (focus on prevention of infection) compared with that for herds with confirmed infection (focus on control of infection). Periodic reassessment is important to compare seroprevalence to the baseline prevalence. It is equally important for periodic evaluation of the management plan and its implementation (e.g., annual risk assessment) by an outside reviewer. For *Salmonella* spp., ongoing evaluation of exposure or fecal shedding may be warranted only if the herd experiences ongoing health problems such as calf mortality (B.P. Smith, DVM, personal communication, 2001).

Facility design and location

Location of adult herd site. Site selection and facility design, as they relate to biosecurity, are important considerations for new dairy start-ups or expanding dairies. In selecting the site and designing facilities, important considerations include drainage, exposure to prevailing winds to optimize natural ventilation, and access roads. In contrast to the swine industry, there are currently no strong recommendations as to minimum distance between dairy or beef farms. It is recommended, however, that animals do not share pasture, water sources, or have fence-line contact with animals from other farms.

Location of youngstock site. The use of segregated production, as with off-site heifer rearing or the use of custom heifer growers to raise replacement animals, is considered important in reducing the risk of exposure and infection of young calves to important pathogens in adult feces. Important pathogens include not only *M. paratuberculosis* and *Salmonella* spp. but also others that cause enteric disease in young calves (e.g., *Escherichia coli*, cryptosporidia, coccidia, rotavirus, and coronavirus; see chapter 2 by Barrington et al.). Because the newborn and young calf are considered to be the most susceptible to infection with *M. paratuberculosis*, early removal from the dam and either segregated or off-site rearing are considered to be important management techniques to reduce the risk for new infection [9,19]. If replacement cattle are raised on the same site, the location of calf hutches, barns, and pastures should be physically isolated from facilities and pastures used for the adult livestock. Manure and feed should be handled in such a way as to prevent youngstock from being exposed to fecal material from older animals, which requires consideration of the manure handling system, the direction of manure flow or drainage, and the equipment used to move feed and manure around the farm. For example, adult manure should not be pushed through or stored in areas (e.g., barnyards) where youngstock have access. Also, manure- or feed-handling equipment contaminated with adult manure should not be allowed to come in contact with youngstock facilities.

Facility design. Whether designing a new facility or retrofitting an old one, careful planning must determine where different groups of animals will be housed; how to achieve adequate ventilation; how to ensure cow and operator comfort and safety; which animal handling and restraint systems to use; and how to determine systems for the flows of vehicles, labor, animals, manure, and feed on the farm. All of these considerations will affect the risk of introduction or transmission of disease on the dairy. The herd veterinarian can become a valuable contributor to the process of helping producers in designing these facilities and in developing written standard operating procedures that determine how various systems function (e.g., traffic, labor, manure, feed, animal flow) and how various tasks are to be performed on the facility.

Facility design for preweaned calves and replacement heifers. Newborn calves should be removed from the dam's environment as soon as possible after birth to prevent exposure to *M. paratuberculosis* and *Salmonella* spp. and other pathogens (cryptosporidia, rotavirus, coronavirus, *E. coli*, and coccidia) in the maternity pen environment. Calves should be processed immediately (colostrum, dip navels, vitamin injections, and so forth) and then quickly placed in calf housing that is physically removed from the adult herd. In the winter months in cold environments, calves may need to be placed first in a calf-warming box or warm room and allowed to dry before placement in hutches or a cold barn. Note that appropriate cleaning and disinfection of these calf-processing and calf-feeding areas need careful attention.

Preweaned calves should be housed individually to minimize opportunities for nose-to-nose contact with pathogens in respiratory secretions and manure from other calves and from older animals. Hutches are ideally suited to this purpose but must be managed to prevent disease transmission between neighboring or successive calves. This management includes selecting or creating a well-drained and well-ventilated site and leaving enough space between hutches to prevent nose-to-nose contact. Hutch placement should be rotated (or alternated) to a new piece of ground between successive calves. The bedding is removed from the old ground, and it is put out to sit, exposed to the sun, for 7 to 14 days. Additionally, hutches should be pressure washed and scrubbed with disinfectant between successive calves. Laying the hutches on their sides with interiors exposed to the sun for 3 to 4 days also helps to kill pathogens. Hutches may not provide sufficient protection for calves against heat stress during the summer. Providing shade over hutches may be necessary to prevent heat stress in particularly hot and humid climates.

Although greenhouse barns and warm barns offer improved operator comfort compared with hutches during the winter months, they are less ideal for the control of infectious disease because ventilation usually is reduced and there is often greater opportunity for direct contact between calves. The postweaning facilities should be designed to allow for easy removal of manure and easy cleaning and disinfecting of both the ground and partitions between successive calves. After weaning, calves should initially be placed in small groups (e.g., 6–10 per pen). In addition to allowing easy delivery of feed, fresh water, and excellent ventilation, these facilities should be designed to allow for easy regular removal of manure and application of fresh bedding as well as easy movement and handling of cattle (e.g., with either a chute or headlock system in place).

Regardless of the housing style selected, producers should look for opportunities to set up the facilities so that calves and youngstock can be moved through different areas (or different age groups) on an "all-in–all-out" basis, similar to that used so successfully in the swine industry. This method allows for complete cleaning and disinfection of facilities before new groups move into the facility, breaking the cycle of disease from old to young. It also minimizes the spread of disease that comes from the "mixing" that occurs when new animals are constantly introduced to an existing group. An all in–all out management system is currently being adopted for calves and replacement heifers by some larger dairies and heifer growers.

Facility design for the adult herd. Whether for a tie-stall or free-stall operation, similar considerations must go into the design of facilities for the adult herd. Areas must be designed for quarantine and processing of new arrivals, far-off dry cows, close-up dry cows, fresh cows, treated and sick cows, and the rest of the milking herd. Sick cows should be housed separately from the rest of the dairy herd (i.e., no nose-to-nose contact or sharing of feed or water). Maternity and fresh cow pens should not be used for sick or lame cows. Drug storage, treatment facilities, and record-keeping systems should be located close to the hospital pen area. All facilities should be designed to allow for the safe and convenient movement, restraint, and treatment of animals, whether a chute system, headlocks, or a management rail system is used.

Maternity pen design and management are of special significance in preventing disease transmission among cows and to the newborn calves. To minimize exposure of the cow and the calf to pathogenic bacteria, the goal must be for the cow to calve into a clean, dry, and well-bedded environment. Because of labor and facility constraints, many herds, both small and large, house and calve dry cows in a group pen and on a bedded pack. Successful management of bedded packs can be achieved only by frequently removing contaminated bedding with liberal and frequent application of fresh bedding. If not extremely well managed, the result is a moist, dirty environment that predisposes cows to infectious diseases such as metritis and mastitis and the newborn calves to umbilical infections and fecal-oral transmission of *M. paratuberculosis*, *Salmonella* spp., and other pathogens (cryptosporidia, rotavirus, coronavirus, *E. coli*, and coccidia). The lack of continuous sunlight exposure in these housing environments prevents ultraviolet light inactivation of pathogens. Not only is the highly susceptible newborn calf exposed to the pathogens from its own dam but also to the pathogens excreted in the manure from all of the dams that have previously been or are currently housed in the same pen.

An alternative to group housing and calving on a bedded pack is the creation of individual maternity pens that are cleaned, disinfected, and rebedded between individual calvings. This model comes closer to the model for farrowing sows, wherein sows farrow in individual crates that are cleaned and disinfected between uses. The system requires herd workers to monitor close-up cows frequently and move individual cows into an individual maternity pen when calving is imminent. The calf and the dam are removed from the pen shortly after delivery, and the area is cleaned, disinfected, and prepared for the next cow. Calves should not be allowed to nurse, and the cow's udder should be cleaned before removal of colostrum for calf feeding. Although this maternity system should be most successful in meeting the objective of delivering the calf into a clean, dry environment (and preventing the transmission of Johne's disease and salmonellosis), it requires resources such as sufficient available labor to allow for frequent observation and timely movement of close-up cows, a gate system that allows for the safe and easy transfer of these cows into the maternity pen by a single person, and a manure-handling system that allows for the quick and convenient removal of contaminated bedding.

Introduction of replacement stock

As is the case with swine, the introduction of new cattle into the herd offers the greatest risk for introducing pathogens onto the dairy. This risk can be minimized in herds with stable herd sizes by rearing replacement heifers within a closed-herd system and using semen from reputable firms with good disease control programs to breed all heifers and cows. Even if heifers are reared at a separate facility, preventing their exposure to cattle from other herds during this period maintains a closed-herd system. Maintaining a closed herd also prevents purchasing, boarding, or loaning of calves, cows, or bulls; sharing pastures or fence lines with ruminants from other farms; returning animals to the herd after shows; and transporting cattle in someone else's vehicle without first cleaning and disinfecting it. Although a truly closed herd may not be practical in today's climate of expanding dairies, farms should ultimately try to move toward a closed-herd system as soon as that option becomes feasible.

If new animals are to be introduced to the herd, steps can still be taken to minimize the risks of introducing new diseases. Veterinarians should assist their clientele in developing protocols for selection of cattle to be introduced into the herd and describing the method of introduction. Although this article focuses on gastrointestinal diseases of adult cattle, most of these recommendations are nonspecific and apply to many other diseases of cattle.

Know the herd of origin. The buyer and seller, or their respective veterinarians, should discuss the current (actual, not hypothetical) herd vaccination program, general herd health status, and specific disease history of the herd of origin and of individual cattle considered for purchase. Buyers also should learn about udder health (i.e., somatic cell count data, bulk tank culture results, clinical mastitis records and culture results, examination and palpation of udders and teat ends), other clinical disease records (e.g., diagnosis of salmonellosis or clinical Johne's disease), and the biosecurity, vaccination, and testing program for the herd of origin. Prospective buyers should avoid purchasing replacement animals from unknown sources or those that have been mixed with other cattle before sale. If possible, producers should purchase heifers rather than mature cows because they are easier to quarantine if not yet milking, and because they are less likely to have contagious mastitis infection. For Johne's disease, there is large benefit to selection of cattle from herds enrolled in a status program (Voluntary Johne's Disease Herd Status Program, to be discussed in more detail in the next section).

Testing purchased cattle. When deciding whether to test for a specific disease, one must consider such factors as the risk of disease introduction, the potential economic and health consequences if the disease is introduced, the accuracy of the diagnostic test being considered, the cost of testing, convenience and potential risks associated with testing, timeliness of test results, how the disease is transmitted, and whether there are other effective ways to manage or control the disease if it is introduced (e.g., vaccination or treatment). Although there is no universal consensus on which diseases to test for, those worth considering and that veterinarians should at least discuss with their clientele include bovine viral diarrhea virus (persistent infection), contagious mastitis (i.e., *Staphylococcus aureus*, *Streptococcus agalactiae*, *Mycoplasma bovis*), *Neospora caninum*, bovine leukosis virus, *Salmonella* spp., and *M. paratuberculosis*. Because it takes 3 to 4 weeks to obtain some test results, samples should be collected and submitted on arrival of the animal into the quarantine area. Alternately, animals may be isolated and tested while they are still on the seller's property, before transport.

For Johne's disease, testing individual cattle is of marginal value and may not be a cost-effective activity (see chapter 9 by Smith). Because of the biology of this disease and the imperfect diagnostic tests currently available, ELISA tests only detect approximately 15% of 24-month old-heifers that are infected with *M. paratuberculosis* but still in the early stages of the disease [23]. Under these circumstances, testing individual heifers will not prevent the introduction of Johne's disease; however, by use of herd screening programs, the infection status of the herd of origin can be determined far more accurately than the infection status of a single individual animal. Producers can dramatically lower the risk of introducing a Johne's disease-infected animal by purchasing animals from herds that have screened the herd and are known to be either negative or have a low disease prevalence. Many states have developed herd status programs to document herd infection status (e.g., Voluntary Johne's Disease Herd Status Program for Cattle).

There may be specific cases, such as in an ongoing herd outbreak, when management changes are ineffective, when testing for *Salmonella* spp. is indicated. In most circumstances, however, the authors do not recommend that producers should routinely test new cattle purchases for *Salmonella* spp., unless concerns exist about *S*. Dublin, which is host-adapted for cattle infection with resultant carrier cattle. The routine culturing of feces is time consuming and expensive. Because carriers are relatively uncommon and shedding is intermittent, the value of screening new purchases by fecal culture is questionable. As for serum antibody testing, B.P. Smith (personal communication, 2001) recommends that persistently high antibody titers must be found on two tests performed 60 to 90 days apart to consider a cow as a carrier. This testing schedule may be impractical for most dairy producers. Ultimately, salmonellosis is a disease best controlled through sanitation and other management practices.

General recommendations for introducing new cattle arrivals are as follows:

1. Purchased animals should be transported in a manner that minimizes stress and injury.
2. Animals should be transported in the buyer's own vehicle, which should be cleaned and disinfected before and after transporting cattle. If someone else's vehicle is used, one should be certain it is cleaned and disinfected before use.
3. New arrivals should be housed in a designated quarantine area for 30 days before allowing contact with resident cattle. The quarantine

period serves to protect both populations of cattle. The resident cattle are protected from exposure to new infections until the quarantined new arrivals can be properly tested, vaccinated, and monitored daily for signs of clinical disease. The new arrivals are protected from exposure to diseases present in the resident herd until they are properly vaccinated and have improved specific immunity to those diseases.

4. Quarantine facilities would, ideally, be located on a separate site. Although less ideal, animals may still be successfully quarantined in a different barn on the same site or even in a separate pen in the same barn as resident cattle. Regardless of the facility constraints, the ultimate goal is for quarantined animals not to share the same air space, waterers, or feeders, or have nose-to-nose contact with resident cattle.
5. The practitioner should collect the necessary samples to test for infectious disease status.
6. Cattle should be treated with a medicated footbath on arrival. The feet should be trimmed and examined by a professional hoof trimmer. Trimming equipment should be disinfected between animals.
7. New arrivals should be dewormed and vaccinated while in quarantine, so that their immune status is similar to that of the resident herd.
8. Daily monitoring should be conducted to evaluate the animal's attitude, appetite, fecal consistency, and rectal temperature for signs of clinical disease.
9. The preceding measures may not be possible when purchasing lactating animals. In this situation, it may be possible to quarantine, test, and vaccinate the group of lactating cows while still on the seller's property. On introduction, the newly purchased animals should be grouped separately from the resident milking herd. The possible spread of contagious mastitis should be prevented by using proper milking hygiene, sanitation of milking equipment, and milking the newly purchased cattle last.

On-farm biosecurity programs

Animal management system. Clinically ill cattle pose a major reservoir of infection from *M. paratuberculosis* and *Salmonella* spp. (especially *Salmonella* Typhimurium). It is important to house these cattle away from high-risk cattle (youngstock and recently fresh cattle) and other healthy cattle if possible. It is especially important not to house these clinically ill cattle in or near the maternity pen to avoid exposure of newborn calves to these pathogens.

Manure management system. Because fecal-oral transmission is the most common route of infection for the gastrointestinal diseases of interest discussed herein (*M. paratuberculosis* and *Salmonella* spp.), manure systems must be designed to provide minimal opportunity for fecal contamination of feed and water sources. Regardless of the system in place, manure should be removed regularly and in the direction away from the most susceptible animals (i.e., calves, youngstock, maternity pens). Equipment (e.g., buckets) used to handle manure should not be used to deliver or push up feed to animals. Because *M. paratuberculosis* can survive in the environment (on pastures or in water) for many months, it is recommended that adult cow manure not be spread on pastures where youngstock are allowed to graze. Using manure-handling systems that recycle flush water (e.g., flush freestall barns) represents a risk for exposing the adult herd to pathogens found in feces [11].

Feed management systems. Careful consideration should be given to the types of feeds provided, as well as systems for feed storage, feed delivery, feed bunk design, and feeding management. One feed-related concern is that many wet byproduct and commodity feeds are often contaminated with *Salmonella*. Practices such as pelleting, steam flaking, and roasting can reduce bacterial numbers. *Salmonella* bacteria are killed by heat processing at temperatures of 55°C (131°F) for 1 hour or 60°C (140°F) for 15 to 20 minutes [2].

Commodity loads should be inspected on delivery for visible evidence of spoilage or mold and the presence of animal droppings (e.g., rodents). Purchasing these feeds fresh, on a frequent basis, and mixing feed immediately before feeding may reduce the risk of using contaminated feed. One should rotate stocks, always feeding the oldest feed out first. A new load of feed should not be dumped on top of the remains of the last load. Feed storage bins, silos, commodity sheds, and other feed storage areas should be cleaned out between batches of feed by pressure washing to remove old feed, dust, bird manure and other contaminants, and then allowing ample time to dry before refilling. All feed delivery equipment should be cleaned between deliveries and farms.

All feeds should be inspected routinely for molds or spoiled material, and if spoiled matter is present, the feed should be discarded and not fed to animals. Feed bunks should be cleaned out daily. Rough, porous feed bunks that can harbor pathogens should be resurfaced to make them smooth. Refusals should not be stored more than 24 hours to prevent spoilage. In general, it is not recommended to feed refusals to youngstock. If refusals are fed to youngstock, they should be fed to the oldest heifers to minimize disease transmission to the more susceptible younger cattle [2]. Similarly, forages and concentrates may be contaminated with *Salmonella* spp. by rodents, cats, dogs, birds, or flies. Rodent, bird, and fly control programs should be implemented in feed storage and handling areas and animal housing areas. Access by cats and dogs should not be allowed in feed storage and handling areas.

The location of feed bunks should be such that feed is easily delivered, refusals are easily removed, and the potential for fecal contamination is minimal. For example, as feed is pushed up to cows or heifers in drive-by feeding systems, care should be taken not to use the same blade for pushing up feed as was used for scraping manure, to avoid pushing the feed or the blade through manure in cow transfer alleys, and not to drive on feed with manure-contaminated wheels. Manure-handling equipment should not be used to handle feed.

Water quality and management. Water odor, taste, mineral content, and bacterial content are determined by testing water sources. Water cups, troughs, and tanks should be designed and positioned to minimize opportunities for fecal contamination and to allow for easy and regular cleaning. Similarly, wells, ponds and streams should be protected from fecal contamination. Youngstock should not have access to barnyards, pasture areas, or water sources where adult cattle have access, where adult manure is stored, or where run-off from adult manure may occur [2].

Control traffic onto and within the farm. Infectious disease can be introduced to the farm by fomites such as transport vehicles, rendering vehicles, and visitors' boots and clothing. Additionally, visitors or farm staff can carry disease from diseased to susceptible animals within the facilities. As with the swine industry, visitors should be instructed to make appointments in advance to visit the farm. Additionally, signs should be posted restricting access to livestock and instructing visitors to go directly to the main office on arrival. All visitors should sign a logbook to allow future evaluation of transfer of pathogens in the case of a disease outbreak.

On larger dairies, farm staff may be designated to work only in one area and with one group of animals (e.g., susceptible calves or fresh cows) and do not work in or travel through areas where diseased animals are housed. If employees are required to work with all groups of animals, as is the case on small and mid-sized dairies, they should work with diseased animals only after handling susceptible animals (e.g., young calves, close-up, fresh, and lactating cows). Alternately, they should wash hands, change clothing, and disinfect boots after having handled sick animals before moving to work with groups of healthy or susceptible groups of animals.

The farm management should provide clean boots and coveralls to all visitors who will access animal facilities or feed storage areas. Dressing should occur in an area designed to prevent cross-contamination. Footbaths should be provided for visitors and farm staff members who are moving between different areas of the farm (e.g., sick-cow area, calf area), with adequate fresh water and scrub brushes available to remove organic material from boots before disinfection. Visitors should have access only to those facilities that concern them (e.g., feed delivery, dead stock, milk pick-up) and should be restricted from parlors and barns.

Veterinarians play a critical role in on-farm biosecurity programs. First, a practicing veterinarian is a potential fomite for disease transmission, with particular risk because of movement from farm to farm after exposure to diseased and infectious animals. Second, a veterinarian should serve as a role model for biosecurity on the farm and a catalyst for positive change among herd managers and workers. The veterinarian should arrive on the farm with clean coveralls and boots, generally move from most susceptible cattle groups to diseased cattle groups (evaluating sick cattle last), wash and disinfect boots between cattle groups, and avoid contaminating feedbunks and feed storage areas with boots. Although the potential role of the veterinarian as a fomite for within-herd transmission of disease among groups of cattle may seem small compared with the everyday flow of people and vehicles on the farm, attention to these details may help to motivate biosecure practices by others.

Vehicles and equipment also should have restricted entry to farms. For example, dead stock trucks, dead stock cables, or dead stock truck drivers should not have access close to or within animal housing facilities or feed storage areas. Carcasses should be removed from these facilities as soon as possible and stored in a remote location that has separate access and is not visible to the public. Drivers of rendering or dead stock vehicles picking up carcasses should be educated to travel directly to this area, through a separate access route if possible [2]. All vehicles and equipment (such as foot-trimming equipment) should be washed, disinfected, and dried before arriving on the farm. No vehicles carrying live animals should be allowed on the farm unless the animals are from an approved source. External vehicles removing manure should be washed and disinfected before being allowed on the farm. All vehicles removing manure from the farm should be restricted from animal housing and feed storage or handling areas.

Vaccination. A conditionally approved killed Johne's disease vaccine is available in certain states with state veterinarian approval. Although the efficacy of this vaccine has not been well demonstrated, it is thought to reduce development of clinical Johne's disease (and reduce fecal shedding) but not to prevent infection. Chronic vaccine-site swellings (i.e., brisket) are a frequent side effect, and accidental inoculation of humans can similarly result in disfiguring lesions. Because the vaccine can be given to calves only up to 35 days of age, vaccination does not lead to immediate herd immunity. Killed *Salmonella* calf vaccines have not proven efficacious [18], but a modified live *S.* Dublin vaccine has been shown to be beneficial when given to young calves (B.P. Smith, DVM, personal communication, 2001). Some benefit may result from vaccination against Johne's disease and salmonellosis in certain situations, but only as an adjunct to the more important biosecurity system in place.

Risk communication

A biosecurity management plan is only as good as its implementation, and any biosecurity system designed for a specific purpose is only as effective as the people who control and manage it. The best management systems can be overwhelmed by human error. All farm workers involved in implementation of the biosecurity plan need to understand its importance to ensure follow-through of the program. Acceptance by the farm's vendors and suppliers, as well as family members and friends, is necessary. For these reasons, it is critical that the herd biosecurity plan be communicated to these individuals clearly, frequently, and consistently.

Biosecurity conclusions

The inability to control diseases such as Johne's disease relying solely on testing and culling has been frustrating. The development of management-related biosecurity programs and systems while evaluating effects on production must be considered. As new research into the diagnosis and control of infectious diseases of cattle is developed, the system will have to adapt as well. It is imperative that cattle producers be forward thinking and open to perspectives from other livestock species (e.g., swine) and implement specific strategies when warranted. Bovine practitioners are in the ideal position to lead the process of re-educating the cattle industry concerning the importance of animal and public health. In so doing, veterinarians must continue to develop novel creative strategies to understand the disease process, to control its spread, and ultimately, to minimize its effect.

References

[1] Akkina J, Angulo F, Hogue, A, et al. *Salmonella typhimurium* DT104 situation assessment. Ft. Collins (CO): USDA-APHIS and USDA-FSIS; 1997. p. 3–7.
[2] Bovine Alliance for Management and Nutrition. Biosecurity of dairy farm feedstuffs. Arlington (VA): BAMN Publications; 2000. p. 1–5.
[3] Buchanan R. Principles of risk assessment for illness caused by foodborne biological agents. Journal of Food Protection 1998;61:1071–74.
[4] Centers for Epidemiology and Animal Health, USDA. Animal and Plant Health Inspection Service: Veterinary Services: Johne's disease on U.S. dairy operations. Publication no. n245.1097. Fort Collins (CO): National Animal Health Monitoring System, 1997. p. 1–52.
[5] Chiodini RJ, Van Kruiningen HJ, Merkal RS. Ruminant paratuberculosis (Johne's disease): the current status and future prospects. Cornell Vet 1984;74:218–62.
[6] Dargatz DA, Byrum BA, Hennager SG, et al. Prevalence of antibodies against *Mycobacterium avium* subsp. *paratuberculosis* among beef cow-calf herds. J Am Vet Med Assoc 2001;219:497–501.
[7] Gay JM, Hunsaker ME. Isolation of multiple *Salmonella* serovars from a dairy two years after a clinical salmonellosis outbreak. J Am Vet Med Assoc 1993;203:1314–20.
[8] Goodger WJ, Collins MT, Nordlund KV, Eisele C, Pelletier J, Thomas CB, et al. Epidemiologic study of on-farm management practices associated with prevalence of *Mycobacterium paratuberculosis* infections in dairy cattle. J Am Vet Med Assoc 1996;208:1877–81.
[9] Groenendaal H, Galligan D. Economical consequences of Johne's disease control programs [doctoral thesis]. New Bolton Center, University of Pennsylvania, Center of Animal Health and Productivity, School of Veterinary Medicine; 1999. p. 1–53.
[10] Hansen LB. Consequences of selection for milk yield from a geneticist's viewpoint. J Dairy Sci 2000;83:1145–50.

[11] Kabagambe EK, Wells SJ, Garber LP, Salman MD, Wagner B, Fedorka-Cray PJ. Risk factors for fecal shedding of *Salmonella* in 91 US dairy herds in 1996. Prev Vet Med 2000;43:177–94.

[12] Kinde H, Read DH, Ardans A, Breitmeyer RE, Willoughby D, Little HE, et al. Sewage effluent: Likely source of *Salmonella enteriditis*, phage type 4 infection in a commercial chicken layer flock in Southern California. Avian Dis 1996;40:672–76.

[13] Larson AB, Merkal RS, Cutlip RC. Age of cattle as related to resistance to infection with *Mycobacterium paratuberculosis*. Am J Vet Res 1975;36:255–57.

[14] Mitscherlich E, Martin EH. *Mycobacterium paratuberculosis*: Microbial survival in the environment. New York: Springer-Verlag; 1984. p. 248–50.

[15] Moore C. Biosecurity and minimal disease. Vet Clin North Am Food Anim Pract 1992;8: 461–74.

[16] Ott SL, Wells SJ, Wagner BA. Herd-level economic losses associated with Johne's disease on U.S. dairy operations. Prev Vet Med 1999;40:179–92.

[17] Radostits OM, Gay CC, Blood DC, Hinchcliff KW. Diseases caused by *Salmonella* spp. In: Veterinary medicine: a textbook of the diseases of cattle, sheep, pigs, goats, and horses, 9th edition. London: WB Saunders; 2000. p. 809–27.

[18] Smith BP. Salmonellosis in ruminants. In: Large animal internal medicine, 3rd edition. St. Louis: Mosby; 2002. p. 775–9.

[19] Smith DR. Biosecurity risk management to improve heifer health and value. In: Proceedings of the Third Annual Professional Dairy Heifer Grower's Association National Conference. March 1999. Bloomington (MN): Professional Dairy Grower's Association; 1999. p. 87–92.

[20] Smith BP, House J. Prospects for *Salmonella* control in cattle. In: Proceedings of the 25th Annual Meeting of the American Association of Bovine Practitioners. St. Paul (MN): AABP; 1992. p. 67–73.

[21] Smith BP, DaRoden L, Thurmond MC, Dilling GW, Konrad H, Patten JA, et al. Prevalence of salmonellae in cattle and in the environment on California dairies. J Am Vet Med Assoc 1994;205:467–71.

[22] Sweeney RW. Transmission of paratuberculosis. Vet Clin North Am Food Anim Pract 1996;12:305–12.

[23] Sweeney RW, Whitlock RH, Buckley CL, Spencer PA. Evaluation of a commercial enzyme-linked immunosorbant assay for the diagnosis of paratuberculosis in dairy cattle. J Vet Diagn Invest 1995;7:488–93.

[24] US Animal Health Association. Foreign animal diseases. Richmond (VA): Committee on Foreign Animal Diseases of the US Animal Health Association, 1998.

[25] Warnick LD, Crofton LM, Pelzer KD, Hawkins MJ. Risk factors for clinical salmonellosis in Virginia, USA cattle herds. Prev Vet Med 2001;49:259–75.

[26] Wells SJ. Biosecurity on dairy operations: Hazards and risks. J Dairy Sci 2000;83:1–7.

[27] Wells SJ, Wagner BA. Herd-level risk factors for infection with *Mycobacterium paratuberculosis* in U.S. dairies and association between familiarity of the herd manager with the disease or prior diagnosis of the disease in the herd and use of preventive measures. J Am Vet Med Assoc 2000;216:1450–57.

[28] Wells SJ, Fedorka-Cray PJ, Dargatz DA, Ferris K, Green A. Fecal shedding of *Salmonella* spp. by dairy cows on-farm and at cull cow markets. J Food Prot 2001;64:3–11.

[29] Wells SJ, Ott SL, Seitzinger AH. Key health concerns for dairy cattle—new and old. J Dairy Sci 1998;81:3029–35.

Appendix

Biosecurity principles for swine populations (Scott Dee, DVM, PhD)

Several important principles are designed to reduce the risk of pathogen introduction to and among naive swine farms: (1) the health status of breeding stock, (2) facility design and location, (3) replacement stock introduction, and (4) on-farm biosecurity programs.

Health status of breeding stock

A proper start to any swine project consists of selecting a breeding stock source that commands the highest level of health. In today's modern swine industry, breeding stock should be free of the following pathogens: porcine reproductive and respiratory syndrome virus, pseudorabies virus, transmissible gastroenteritis virus, swine influenza virus H1N1/H3N2, porcine circovirus type 2, *Brucella suis*, *Mycoplasma hyopneumoniae*, *Actinobacillus pleuropneumoniae*, toxigenic *Pasteurella multocida* type D, *Serpulina hyodysenteriae*, *Salmonella choleraesuis*, and *Sarcoptes suis*. Selection of the source herd should follow a careful review of diagnostic and production data and communication with a staff veterinarian. A monitoring program should be in place within the source herd, and testing should take place monthly by the collection of a representative sample of each pig population using both antibody and antigen tests when available. Proper sample sizes should be calculated according to population size, the desired level of confidence of the sampling protocol, and the sensitivity and specificity of each test used. Diagnostic evaluation of tissues collected from clinically abnormal pigs should be conducted on a routine basis, and records made available at all times. A thorough understanding of the health status of the seedstock source minimizes the risk of introducing unwanted pathogens into a herd. Proper planning includes communication and sharing of diagnostic data between veterinarians and producers before purchase.

Facility design and location

The risks of contracting an infectious disease are much higher in extremely hog-dense areas, so construction of new facilities should always initially focus on site location. A minimum of 2 miles (3.2 km) is suggested between farms, although little scientific data are available to support this claim. The use of segregated production is also important to minimize the spread of pathogens between animal populations and to interrupt the cycle of pathogens that occur from older to younger pigs. Segregated production involves the rearing of weaned and growing pigs on sites separate from the sow herd. Segregated production techniques, although ideally requiring separate sites, can be practiced on a single site, so long as the weaned-pig facility is separate from the sow herd. Functional distances for on-site segregation range from 50 to 100 yards (Scott Dee, DVM, PhD, personal experience, 1993–2001).

Replacement stock introduction

The largest risk of pathogen entry to a swine farm is through the introduction of replacement breeding stock, so many producers have adapted programs to raise their replacement females using a closed-herd system. Internal multiplication of breeding stock is an effective way to minimize the risk of pathogen introduction to a farm and often results in consistent exposure of growing pigs to farm-specific microflora, a practice which frequently improves overall herd immunity. If such a practice is not possible, all incoming replacement gilts from an external source should be quarantined, blood-tested to ensure the proper health status, and then acclimated to farm-specific microflora before entry. The quarantine facility should ideally be located on a separate site, away from the sow herd. The facility should use all in–all out animal flow, and producers should care for these animals after leaving the sow herd for the day. Animals should be blood-tested on arrival and 1 week before entry to the sow farm to ensure that the desired health status has been maintained throughout the quarantine period.

On-farm biosecurity programs

Moore [15] has written a comprehensive review on the biosecurity of swine units, and readers should refer to it for additonal detail. To minimize disease transmission, breeding should be done by artificial insemination (AI). Semen should be purchased from a reputable AI center with a documented high-quality health status monitored on a monthly basis. Semen should be distributed by a courier service to neutral delivery points located at the perimeter of the farm. Other biosecurity measures include a minimum of 48 hours free of swine contact and shower facilities for all personnel before entry into the sow and boar centers. Fumigation rooms are an excellent way to disinfect inanimate objects, such as tools and feed bags, before their entry into the animal airspace. For personnel movement between on-site facilities, personnel should change boots and coveralls and wash their hands before entering each facility. Professional exterminators should be hired on a contract basis to visit farms monthly. All openings to facilities should be bird-proofed, using bird screen, particularly over the sidewall openings to naturally ventilated finishing facilities. Other important components of a sound biosecurity program include incineration of carcasses, washing and disinfecting transport vehicles when marketing animals, and perimeter fencing.

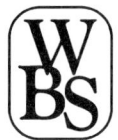

THE VETERINARY
CLINICS
Food Animal
Practice

Vet Clin Food Anim 18 (2002) 57–77

Biosecurity and bovine respiratory disease

Robert J. Callan, DVM, PhD*,
Franklyn B. Garry, DVM, MS

*Department of Clinical Sciences, College of Veterinary Medicine and Biomedical Sciences,
Colorado State University, 300 West Drake Road, Fort Collins, CO 80523, USA*

Respiratory disease problems represent a major area of concern for all phases of cattle production. All types and all ages of cattle are susceptible to respiratory problems, and in some production settings, respiratory disease is the single most important cause of livestock morbidity and mortality. In recent national surveys, respiratory disease is reported to account for 24.5% of preweaned dairy heifer calf deaths, and it is the leading cause of death in weaned heifer calves, accounting for 44.8% of calf death losses [54]. In adult dairy cows, respiratory disease is less important than mastitis, lameness, metabolic diseases, and reproductive disorders as a cause of morbidity, but it still affects 2.5% of adult dairy cattle on a yearly basis, and 9.6% of dairy cow deaths are attributed to respiratory disease [54]. In preweaned beef calves over 3 weeks of age, respiratory problems represent 21% of health problems, occurring in approximately 0.8% of all calves [52]. Respiratory disease accounts for 16.3% of total beef calf death loss and 6.0% of total breeding cattle death loss on cow–calf operations [52]. Shipping fever was recently reported to occur in 14.4% of feedlot cattle, and this respiratory problem was more than 4 times more prevalent than the next leading cause of morbidity, which was acute interstitial pneumonia [56]. Annual death loss estimates due to respiratory disease for all cattle and calves in the United States exceed 1.2 million animals, with an estimated total economic loss greater than $478 million [53].

These morbidity and mortality estimates underscore the tremendous importance of respiratory disease to cattle producers. Considerable effort over many years has been focused on improving our understanding of this problem. Despite improvements in our understanding of pathogenesis, characteristics of causative agents, vaccine technology, and means of prevention

---

* Corresponding author.
E-mail address: rcallan@colostate.edu (R.J. Callan).

and treatment, it seems that respiratory disease remains one of the foremost cattle health concerns.

The challenge that the authors were presented with in writing this article was to consider the role that biosecurity could play in reducing the occurrence or effect of respiratory disease. It seems that little research has specifically evaluated the effects of biosecurity management practices on the occurrence of the problem in livestock operations. Indeed, recognizing the multifactorial etiology of infectious respiratory disease and the ubiquitous presence of the pathogens involved leads to the conclusion that attempts to decrease disease prevalence must incorporate multiple management steps, of which biosecurity practices are only a single component. Although biosecurity practices have equal potential to decrease respiratory disease losses in all food animal species, the authors focus this article primarily on bovine respiratory disease complex. This article addresses major areas of respiratory pathogen control and provides some suggestions for practical intervention.

Overview of bovine respiratory disease

Bovine respiratory disease is not a single entity, nor is it attributable to a single cause [2]. One useful scheme for characterizing respiratory tract diseases in a practical manner distinguishes three different categories of problems [40]. These include the bovine respiratory disease complex (BRDC), epitomized by shipping fever pneumonia and enzootic calf pneumonia; acute interstitial pneumonias; and metastatic pneumonia. This scheme excludes many problems that involve only the upper respiratory tract, although these problems may predispose to lower tract infections. The interstitial pneumonias are most commonly attributed to toxicoses, and metastatic pneumonias are secondary complications of disease in other organ systems that spread hematogenously to the lung. Although these disease problems are frequently fatal for affected cattle, they occur sporadically and are generally not considered to be contagious. The authors focus their attention for this discussion on BRDC. This problem has an infectious origin, and it is by far the most frequently occurring form of cattle respiratory disease. Cattle of all ages and in a variety of circumstances can be affected by BRDC, but the disease most commonly manifests in young dairy calves (enzootic calf pneumonia) and in beef calves recently arrived at feedlots (shipping fever pneumonia).

Research over the past several decades has provided an increasingly clear picture of how BRDC occurs and why it is so common. Unfortunately, this knowledge has not led to a commensurate decrease in the morbidity and mortality associated with this problem, primarily because animals are commonly managed in ways that predispose to disease development.

Bovine respiratory disease complex refers to bacterial bronchopneumonia that may or may not be complicated by previous or concurrent viral or

Mycoplasma infection [2]. Numerous bacterial species can be isolated from the lungs of affected animals. In feedlot cattle and adult cattle, *Mannheimia (Pasteurella) haemolytica* is considered the most important pathogen, with lesser roles attributed to *Pasteurella multocida* and *Hemophilus somnus*. In younger calves, these same pathogens play a role, but *Mycoplasma* spp. are also considered to be important. *Arcanobacterium pyogenes, Fusobacterium* spp., and *Bacteroides* spp. are frequently isolated from animals with chronic, abscessing lung lesions but do not play a major role in acute bronchopneumonia. Less common bacterial isolates, including *Streptococcus* spp., *Staphylococcus* spp., *Pseudomonas aeruginosa*, and *Chlamydia* spp., are also occasionally identified in young calves.

All of the bacterial pathogens considered important in BRDC can be isolated from the upper respiratory tract of healthy cattle and calves. These pathogens are considered ubiquitous in cattle populations, not because they can be found in each animal, but because they are readily identified in the nasopharynx of some animals in most populations. In the absence of other predisposing causes of disease, it seems that the simple presence of these bacterial agents is not of major significance. The disease complex is best characterized as being multifactorial, only occurring when a combination of factors involving the animal, environment, and infectious agents are present.

Viral pathogens are implicated in the development of BRDC, although the final pulmonary pathology is primarily caused by bacterial pathogens [2]. The principal viruses involved in BRDC include bovine herpesvirus 1 (infectious bovine rhinotracheitis), bovine parainfluenza virus type 3, bovine respiratory syncytial virus, and bovine viral diarrhea virus. Lesser roles are attributed to bovine coronavirus, adenovirus, rhinovirus, reovirus, and enterovirus. These viral pathogens primarily infect the upper respiratory tract, resulting in rhinitis, tracheitis, and bronchitis. Their ability to cause direct pulmonary disease is generally limited except for bovine respiratory syncytial virus, which can also cause severe lung damage as the primary agent. All of these viral pathogens predispose the lung to bacterial infection and bronchopneumonia. The primary role of these agents in BRDC is to promote bacterial challenge to the lungs by compromising respiratory tract defense mechanisms.

The predisposing causes of BRDC act synergistically and are most commonly identified in combination rather than as single causative problems. The list of predisposing animal factors is long and includes animal age, decreased immune responsiveness due to animal stress, lack of previous viral exposure or vaccination, inadequate passive immunoglobulin transfer in young calves, nutritional deficiencies, and dehydration. Environmental risk factors include high air humidity or dust content, rapidly changing environmental temperatures, extreme heat or cold, and high concentrations of noxious gases such as ammonia. Several risk factors may increase pathogen density or pathogen exposure, although these risk factors probably act by other means as well. For example, commingling cattle from multiple sources may increase exposure to antigenically heterogeneous viral pathogens, while also increasing animal stress. Poor ventilation and high humidity can increase pathogen density and survival time but also can increase noxious gas concentrations and adversely affect pulmonary function. Animal crowding increases airborne pathogen exposure but also induces animal stress and reduces immune responsiveness.

Prevention of bovine respiratory disease complex

When evaluating the rate of BRDC occurrence in cattle populations, it is clear that efforts to prevent this disease have not been effective on an industry-wide basis, although some individual producers have successfully used prevention strategies. The two biggest areas of BRDC effect are in the form of enzootic calf pneumonia of dairy calves and shipping fever pneumonia of feedlot cattle. Given our current understanding of this disease problem, it is clear that the animal management systems employed for these groups of animals (i.e., dairy calf–rearing systems and feedlot cattle–receiving systems) have failed to rigorously apply knowledge of disease pathogenesis and prevention into their processes. This situation may be changing currently, as the beef production industry increasingly uses quality-assurance principles in production systems and develops marketing procedures and animal-purchasing practices that reward improvements in animal health [12,35,46]. Similarly, the dairy industry has begun to recognize the economic benefit of improved calf health and increasingly uses specialized calf-rearing systems [1,44].

Because the purpose of this article is to examine the role of biosecurity management in respiratory disease prevention, the authors do not attempt to provide a complete review of BRDC preventive practices. Many of the important means of preventing BRDC do not employ biosecurity but are targeted toward enhancing animal immune preparedness and enhancing animal response to infectious challenge. Effective respiratory disease preventive practices are those targeted at reducing identified risk factors for disease development [1,2,35,46]. These practices include management to improve animal nutrition with special emphasis on micronutrient nutrition, practices that reduce animal stress, reduced commingling of animals, improved animal transportation and feedlot receiving practices, improved preconditioning and vaccination programs that emphasize vaccination before shipment and during times of low calf stress, and improved ventilation with reduced crowding.

It is important to consider the factors that drive the development and implementation of disease prevention and biosecurity programs. The most apparent of these factors is the effect on animal production and growth; however, all interventions have their cost, and these costs must always be considered relative to the potential economic returns. Unfortunately, information regarding the financial impact of herd biosecurity programs is limited, and estimates based on clinical experience must often be applied. Other issues, including herd pathogen status and its effect on livestock marketing, food product quality assurance, drug residues, injection site lesions, antimicrobial resistance, and animal welfare also contribute to the forces that drive the development of biosecurity programs. Ultimately, a biosecurity program must be integrated into the overall herd management. It must be developed using a team approach that addresses the concerns of the producer, the economic effect on the production unit, the influence on product quality, and public health concerns. The veterinarian is best suited to effectively develop and implement such programs.

The multifactorial nature of BRDC and the ubiquitous presence of respiratory pathogens are important concepts when considering the role that biosecurity can play in decreasing the prevalence of disease. For infectious diseases in which point source pathogen exposure, high susceptibility, and high virulence are prominent features of disease transmission (e.g., anthrax, foot-and-mouth disease, rabies, and so forth), limiting animal contact with the pathogen is a key feature of disease prevention and may even provide the means of disease eradication. Alternatively, when the causative pathogens are endemic in a population and individual susceptibility is dependent on numerous interrelated factors, the management of animal resistance and risk factors may be proportionally more important for disease prevention than biosecurity practices. It appears that BRDC prevention requires a combination of management to enhance animal resistance plus management to reduce exposure to the pathogens. The important point is not to de-emphasize the value of reducing pathogen introduction, exposure, and transmission (i.e., biosecurity) but to also stress the importance of other management features that promote animal resistance. It is particularly important that preventive management practices be coordinated and used in combination, because no single management procedure will be successful without the complement of other practices. It is likely that our inability to reduce the prevalence of respiratory disease in cattle is, in part, attributable to our failure to integrate multiple aspects of respiratory disease prevention practices, including biosecurity.

The fundamental concept of biosecurity is to decrease pathogen transmission between animals. Transmission of respiratory pathogens occurs by close nose-to-nose contact, environmental or fomite exposure, and airborne exposure. Increased contact between shedding and susceptible individuals increases pathogen spread. Environmental exposure through common areas and equipment that involve oral or nasal contact such as feed bunks, water troughs, and salt blocks may be an even greater risk, however.

Total environmental pathogen load is extremely important in considering respiratory pathogen transmission. Environmental contamination from animals in contact is the primary source of most respiratory pathogens. Individual animal shedding is quite variable and depends on the etiologic agent, the time course of the disease, the clinical severity, and the immune response of the host. In general, clinically ill animals shed greater numbers of pathogens than normal or asymptomatic animals; however, it must be recognized that individuals periodically shed both viral and bacterial respiratory pathogens without evidence of disease. Well-vaccinated animals may also periodically shed pathogens and should not necessarily be considered completely safe from disease transmission.

The persistence of the pathogen in the environment also contributes to pathogen exposure. Environmental pathogen survival times depend on many factors, including organic material, moisture, direct sunlight, and exposure to disinfectants. Environmental survival times for most viral respiratory pathogens are probably on the order of minutes to several hours [18,47]. Survival times for bacterial pathogens may be longer depending on the environmental conditions and the organism. Airborne transmission is dependent on numerous factors, including ambient temperature, relative humidity, airborne particle (dust) density, ventilation, prevailing wind, and structural or geographic obstructions [47]. Airborne transmission of typical viral respiratory pathogens can occur over distances as far as 4 meters and possibly further [29,30]. Airborne transmission of other viruses such as foot-and-mouth disease virus or pseudorabies virus has been shown to occur over many miles, however [10,11,15,45,47]. Adding to the complexity of pathogen transmission, it seems that the efficiency of transmission is different between different strains of a given pathogen [30]. Understanding how management practices can reduce either pathogen shedding or exposure is the key to creating effective biosecurity programs.

Biosecurity and bovine respiratory disease complex

The term *biosecurity* is used for those management and hygiene practices that reduce introduction, exposure, and transmission of infectious agents. Although biosecurity may not provide the single most important component of respiratory disease prevention, reducing pathogen exposure is a valuable part of any infectious disease management system. Little information is available to specifically evaluate the effect of individual biosecurity practices in prevention of BRDC, but there are some important respiratory disease prevention practices that limit pathogen exposure and good reason to more closely evaluate the role that biosecurity could play in the future. The authors emphasize five areas of biosecurity management that should be more rigorously applied for the reduction of respiratory disease prevalence in cattle, including (1) strategic vaccination, (2) calf biosecurity, (3) housing ventilation, (4) commingling and animal contact, and (5) bovine viral diarrhea virus control.

Strategic vaccination

Many improvements in vaccine technology have occurred over the past few decades, and practitioners have an array of improved bovine respiratory pathogen vaccines at their disposal [35]. Unfortunately, the current respiratory pathogen vaccines have not all been scrutinized for efficacy to the most desirable degree, and many do not protect against respiratory disease nearly as effectively as some veterinarians and producers would like to believe. Although vaccines directed at specific conserved proteins, such as toxoid vaccines, may completely prevent a particular disease, vaccines against complex disease agents that have multiple antigenic strains are unlikely to be capable of such levels of protection. Respiratory vaccines are better viewed as disease modifiers than absolute preventive agents.

Vaccines are usually used as a means to decrease the likelihood or severity of disease occurrence in the individual animal receiving the vaccination. Indeed, vaccine efficacy may be evaluated in many ways, but the more rigorous evaluations involve the ability of a vaccinated animal to withstand a challenge of disease or pathogen exposure [42]. Practitioners tend to view vaccination as one of the management factors that enhance animal resistance to infection and thus augment the value of biosecurity management by working to reduce susceptibility to infectious disease rather than decrease exposure and transmission. For respiratory disease prevention, however, effective vaccination can also serve as part of a biosecurity management system. In addition to preventing disease, a vaccine's efficacy might also be considered for its ability to limit pathogen shedding when infection does occur. Vaccine-induced immunity often results in decreased magnitude and duration of pathogen shedding [6,16,59]. Because exposure is directly related to pathogen concentration in the environment, it follows that vaccine-induced reductions in shedding should decrease transmission within a susceptible population.

Proper vaccine use and a well-managed vaccination program can be viewed as part of a complete biosecurity program. At a minimum, a good vaccination program should include the following:

- Proper storage and administration of the vaccine as indicated by the manufacturer's labeled recommendations.
- Vaccination of all susceptible animals, including both resident and incoming animals.
- Application of the vaccine to systemically healthy, well-nourished, minimally stressed, and immunocompetent cattle.
- Strategic timing of vaccination so that it precedes contact with new animals long enough to allow an appropriate immune response.
- Revaccination as recommended for the particular vaccine product.

Calf biosecurity

Biosecurity management of calves is extremely important for development of healthy animals. Many of the biosecurity recommendations for newborn calves focus on decreasing the transmission of enteric pathogens; however, these same principles can be important for minimizing respiratory disease problems. Several details of calf biosecurity management deserve emphasis.

Environmental and housing factors significantly affect calf health and viability. Differences in calf management for cow–calf herds versus dairies are related to the relative risk of respiratory disease between these two production groups. Beef calves are generally raised in open-range situations that effectively dilute the exposure to respiratory pathogens. Although beef calves are continually exposed to pathogens shed from adult cattle and other calves, the magnitude of pathogen exposure before weaning is generally low, resulting in relatively little respiratory disease. In contrast to many enteric pathogens, the environmental survival time of the respiratory pathogens is limited [18], and accumulation of pathogens in the environment is not considered a primary concern.

Dairy calf housing has a significant effect on the incidence of respiratory disease in neonatal calves. Although the common viral respiratory pathogens can be transmitted over distances up to 4 meters [29,30], properly spaced calf hutches seem to effectively limit aerosol transmission of respiratory pathogens. The short survival of these pathogens in the environment limits the transmission between successive occupants of an individual hutch. Disinfection procedures that are used for enteric diseases should be more than sufficient to decrease respiratory pathogen transmission (see article by Barrington et al. in this issue). In contrast, there is a high risk of respiratory disease transmission in group-raised neonatal calves. Factors including the number of animals, relative animal density, housing facilities, and ventilation conditions significantly contribute to transmission in grouped calves and are discussed in subsequent sections of this article.

Numerous management practices can decrease exposure and transmission of respiratory pathogens to calves in dairy operations. Feeding pasteurized milk or milk replacer is a useful biosecurity practice for minimizing the spread of enteric agents such as *Salmonella* spp. or *Mycobacterium avium* subsp. *paratuberculosis.* These practices are also effective at limiting ingestion of potential respiratory pathogens. *Mycoplasma* spp. bacteria are commonly implicated in newborn calf disease, including enzootic calf pneumonia [2,37,48,49]. Although *Mycoplasma* spp. may spread by the airborne route, it is also a common mastitis pathogen and can be shed from clinically or subclinically infected cows [24,37,49]. Nasopharyngeal colonization occurs after oral ingestion of contaminated milk, potentially resulting in clinical respiratory disease in calves [37]. *Mycoplasma* spp. and other pathogens can also spread hematogenously after ingestion by a susceptible calf [24,37]. Similarly, other potential respiratory pathogens such as *Streptococcus* spp., *Staphylococcus* spp., *Salmonella* spp., and *Escherichia coli* can be recovered from milk and spread hematogenously to the lungs after oral ingestion. Bovine viral diarrhea virus is shed in the milk of persistently infected cattle. Ingestion of bovine viral diarrhea virus–contaminated milk can result in respiratory and systemic infections, possible immune suppression, and respiratory disease.

Proper cleaning and disinfection of calf feeding equipment, including nursing bottles, buckets, and mixing utensils, should be performed. Equipment should be cleaned with a detergent and disinfected between uses. A common and economical disinfectant is standard household bleach used at a 1:10 dilution. Bottles and equipment that are potentially shared between multiple animals should be soaked for 15 to 20 minutes in this solution. Although bleach will not completely kill all potential pathogens, it is effective at significantly decreasing viable numbers and thus contributing to decreased exposure and transmission between feedings.

Prompt removal of dairy calves from the maternity pen environment, where they are exposed to numerous adult cow pathogens, can also decrease transmission of potential respiratory pathogens. Newborn calves should not have direct contact with older calves and adults. Calf hutch spacing should be evaluated, with a minimum of 4 feet of separation between calves. Worker hygiene can minimize contamination of calf feed and the calf environment. Appropriate vaccination of dams before colostral production can increase passive transfer of effective antibodies, reducing the risk of exposure and potential shedding after infection. It has been demonstrated that good colostral transfer to beef calves was associated with decreased occurrence of disease episodes and improved calf performance all the way through the growing and finishing period in feedlot animals [36]. It is unlikely that the passive transfer of immunoglobulins per se is specifically responsible for beneficial effects on the long-term health of animals, but profound effects may result from management that improves newborn health and disease resistance. This in turn provides for improved nutrition, growth, physiologic well-being, and decreased total pathogen load.

Numerous calfhood husbandry procedures should be considered as standard biosecurity protocols for all infectious diseases, including respiratory disease. Sick animals should be identified and separated from healthy animals. A specific calf-isolation area should be established, with consideration to animal comfort and ease of cleaning and disinfection. Where practical, individual equipment should be used for each separate calf. Specific care and treatment personnel should be identified, and animals with suspected infectious diseases should be treated after handling healthy animals. Additional personnel hygiene protocols include dedicated coveralls to be used in the sick pens, the use of rubber overboots, and disinfectant footbaths. Personnel should be encouraged to wash their hands before and after entering the sick pens and between caring for animals with dissimilar disease conditions. In many cases, equipment and facilities need to be made available to help establish such procedures.

Similar biosecurity management practices can be used in cow–calf herds. Although feeding pasteurized milk or milk replacer is obviously not a practical management practice, milk-borne exposure to pathogens can be minimized by proper attention to the adult cows. Adult cattle must be appropriately vaccinated to provide optimal colostral immunity to the calves and to decrease adult cow infections and shedding. Adult cow nutrition should be optimized to improve colostrum quality. Adult cow nutrition can also have a dramatic effect on calving ease and decrease the incidence of dystocia. Special attention should be placed on high-risk calves, including calves delivered with manual assistance, cesarean section, born in inclement weather, weak or premature calves, and multiple births. Such calves often do not nurse colostrum in a timely fashion or have impaired absorption of immunoglobulin. Cows should be evaluated for evidence of clinical mastitis and treated or culled as appropriate. Decreased morbidity can be observed by minimizing the time that beef cow–calf pairs spend in a designated calving area, where pathogen loads tend to increase throughout the calving season. Bovine viral diarrhea virus surveillance and eradication in cows and calves should also be used (see discussion in a following section).

As can be seen from the preceding discussion, many of the management practices that contribute to biosecurity of respiratory disease are standard quality-assurance practices that are recommended for basic calf health.

Ventilation

Good ventilation is a critical aspect of animal management and can profoundly affect respiratory health. Several discussions of ventilation and its effect on animal health are present in the literature [2–5,13,14,19,27,31, 34,38,39,43,51,58]. Proper ventilation serves eight primary functions:

1. It decreases the airborne pathogen concentration
2. It eliminates noxious gases (ammonia, hydrogen sulfide, carbon dioxide, carbon monoxide, and methane)
3. It decreases airborne dust contamination
4. It decreases airborne endotoxin levels
5. It maintains optimum ambient temperature
6. It maintains optimum environmental humidity levels
7. It eliminates drafts
8. It eliminates areas of stagnant air

With respect to biosecurity, one of the most important aspects of proper ventilation is the reduction in the concentration of airborne pathogens. All of the important viral and bacterial respiratory pathogens can spread aerogenously and can attain high concentrations in poorly ventilated housing areas. Airborne pathogen concentration is a function of many factors, including animal type, housing system, stocking rate, bedding, humidity, dust particle density and size, and finally, elimination through ventilation. Improved ventilation is one important means whereby airborne pathogen concentration can be readily decreased within the given constraints of an operation; however, pathogen removal is not a linear function, and practical and theoretical limits are often observed [33]. Studies of building ventilation for humans demonstrate potential reductions in airborne exposure of pathogens and disease incidence, although improved ventilation beyond that which provides comfort may not be practical or provide significant additional benefit [33]. As the airborne pathogen load rises, ventilation provides progressively less protection against respiratory infections. It is important to realize that stocking rate has a more dramatic effect on airborne pathogen density than ventilation [33,58]. For example, a two-fold increase in stocking rate requires nearly a 10-fold increase in ventilation to maintain the same airborne pathogen density [58]. Ventilation cannot overcome grossly inadequate housing, management, or hygiene within a production unit.

Along with stocking density, there are other practical concerns that contribute to airborne pathogen density and transmission. One of these is related to animal handling and excitement. It is extremely important to handle grouped animals in a calm environment with minimal animal activity and stress. Increased animal activity not only increases dust exposure (which contains airborne pathogens) but also increases ventilatory rate, ventilatory effort, and tidal volume, which in turn increases the amount of aerosolized pathogen shed by infected animals and the amount of pathogen inhaled by susceptible animals. The increased dust exposure will also adversely affect mucociliary clearance and respiratory defense mechanisms.

Part of the effect of ventilation is to minimize airborne contaminants that can impair respiratory function and defense mechanisms [34,38,39,58]. Significant airborne contaminants include ammonia, hydrogen sulfide, carbon dioxide, carbon monoxide, methane, dust particles, and endotoxin. Ammonia and hydrogen sulfide are toxic gases and can contribute to respiratory damage, decreased mucociliary clearance, decreased alveolar macrophage activity, and overall compromise to respiratory defense mechanisms. Carbon dioxide, carbon monoxide, and methane contribute primarily as asphyxiative gases and generally do not contribute to significant impairment of the respiratory tract.

Dust particles also contribute to the impairment of respiratory defense mechanisms. Dust particles can arise from both organic and inorganic sources. In general, particles greater than 5 μm are filtered out by the nasal passages; most particles from 2 to 5 μm are removed by the mucociliary clearance of the trachea and bronchi, and particles less than 2 μm can penetrate to the alveolar spaces [47,58]. Organic and inorganic dust particles can impair mucociliary clearance and overload alveolar macrophage phagocytic clearance [58]. Organic dust particles are generally of more concern in confinement and intensive housing situations. In animal housing environments, most of the organic dust arises from fecal material, skin, and hair. Organic dust is significant in that it often contains high endotoxin and pathogen levels [38,39]. Inhaled endotoxin can contribute to pulmonary compromise by initiating inflammatory reactions within the alveoli and alveolar vascular endothelium.

Appropriate ventilation is also important in maintaining acceptable humidity and ambient temperature levels within confinement or semi-open housing. Observed thermoneutral ranges (the range of air temperature that sustains optimal performance) for a variety of domestic livestock are available (Table 1) [58]. In general, livestock can perform adequately within a fairly wide thermoneutral range. Higher temperatures, especially when combined with high humidity, tend to be more problematic than low temperatures [34]. Depending on the given climate and temperature ranges of a geographic region, housing ventilation will need to be designed to provide either heating or cooling or both. Cold temperatures and perhaps temperature fluctuations can decrease mucociliary clearance and predispose animals to respiratory disease [17]. Often, wide temperature fluctuations are more detrimental to animal health because they do not allow suitable adaptation over time.

There is minimal information on how ambient temperature directly relates to airborne pathogen biosecurity. Increased ambient temperature results in increased respiration and may increase pathogen shedding from infected animals. The direct effects of ambient temperature on pathogen survival are relatively unknown. Some studies suggest that the concentration of airborne particles is increased at low temperatures, and airborne bacterial concentrations were higher in winter than in summer [47].

There is slightly more information concerning the effects of relative humidity on pathogen survival and thus, airborne biosecurity [47,58]. In general, viruses with a hydrophobic lipid outer shell (i.e., enveloped viruses) survive better in lower humidity, and lipid-free viruses (i.e., foot-and-mouth disease virus) are more stable in moist air [18,47]. The four primary viral respiratory pathogens in cattle (bovine herpesvirus 1, bovine parainfluenza virus type 3, bovine respiratory syncytial virus, and bovine viral diarrhea virus) are all enveloped viruses and would be considered more stable in dry air, although

Table 1
Estimated thermoneutral values (°C) for several livestock species and age groups

Livestock group	Minimum acclimated temperature	Minimum ideal temperature	Maximum ideal temperature	Maximum acclimated temperature
Newborn calf	10	10	25	37
1-month-old calf	0	0	25	30
Veal calf	−15	−5	22	30
Beef cows	−17	−10	20	27
Dairy cow	−25	0	22	27
Ewe	−10	−5	25	37
Newborn lamb	20	20	32	37
Growing lamb	−12	0	22	37

From Wathes CM, Jones CD, Webster AJ. Ventilation, air hygiene and animal health. Vet Rec 1983;113:554–9; with permission.

the authors are unaware of specific studies documenting this conclusion. Gram-negative bacteria have outer phospholipid membranes and are also expected to be more stable in dry air [47]. *Mycoplasma* are reported to be sensitive to relative humidity between 40% and 70% [58]. Extrapolation of these limited data suggests that typical airborne pathogens associated with respiratory disease in domestic animals survive better in cool, dry air such as is observed in the late fall, winter, and early spring months. Although this correlates with clinical observations concerning the relative seasonal incidence of respiratory disease, a direct association has not been established. In beef cattle, seasonal increases in respiratory disease also correlate with seasonal management practices associated with movement of cattle to feedlots and increased animal density. It is likely that climate and management factors act together to dramatically increase pathogen exposure and transmission in feedlots. Alternatively, the high humidity that can be observed with dairy confinement housing in cold weather probably contributes to increased respiratory disease because of the higher pathogen density associated with increased aerosolized particle concentrations.

Ventilation systems should be constructed to provide even airflow throughout the structure without areas of air stagnation or drafts. Pockets of air stagnation have higher levels of airborne contaminants and contribute to the exposure and transmission of respiratory pathogens. Air stagnation can often be remedied by appropriate use of inexpensive fans. Correcting draft conditions can be more problematic and often requires complete evaluation of the housing structure for air leaks and evaluation of the ventilation system, especially air intake vents.

Guidelines for housing of livestock have been reported, including recommendations for ventilation (Table 2) [2,5,13,27,34,51,58]. Appropriate ventilation should flow from younger to older animals to minimize spread of pathogens to the more susceptible animals. The total air volume should be completely changed 4 times per hour in winter, and it should be changed up to 30 times per hour in summer [5,51]. The ventilation system should

Table 2
Recommended space requirements for calves

	Confinement housing				
Age of calf (wk)	<6	6–12	12–16		
Air volume (m³/calf)	6	10	15		
	Open housing				
Age of calf (mo)	0–5	5–8	9–12	13–15	16–24
Sheltered area (ft²/calf)	21	25	28	32	40
Outside open area (ft²/calf)	30	35	40	45	50
Total area (ft²/calf)	51	60	68	77	90

Confinement housing *From* Klingborg DJ. Preventing calf pneumonia. Compend Contin Educ Pract Vet 1986;8:F112–14; with permission.

Fundamental recommendations for ventilation systems in confinement and open-sheltered housing

Confinement housing
- Minimum of four air changes per hour (winter)
- Total exhaust capacity for up to 30 air changes per hour (summer)
- Continuous (not intermittent) ventilation
- Single-speed fans, not variable-speed fans, should be used
- Fans must be able to sustain 1/8-inch static pressure
- One must allow for two to four different ventilation rates using multiple fans
- Enough inlet slot area should be provided to allow minimal inlet velocity of 100 fpm (winter) and 800 fpm (summer)
- Thermostats should be used to control ventilation fans
- Thermostats should be located at eye level near the center of the barn
- The ventilation rate should be altered by stepping up the number of fans used for each level
- Wall fans should be mounted near the ceiling but collect air using ducts from within 38 cm (15 in) of the floor
- The fresh air intake should be located near the ceiling but at least 4 feet from any exhaust fan
- Adjustable eave slot inlets should be used to distribute incoming air uniformly
- A system for supplemental heat in the winter should be provided

Open-shelter housing
- Ventilation occurs through both open sides and the roof (ridge ventilation)
- Fully closed ends should be no more than 30 feet wide
- End widths greater than 30 feet require inlet ventilation
- Widths of 60 to 70 feet result in pockets of air stagnation
- The building should be oriented with the long axis perpendicular to the prevailing wind
- Open sides should face away from the prevailing wind
- Ventilation fans should be directed out of the downwind side of the building
- The building should be located upwind of other structures that might block air flow
- One should avoid placing shelter within 75 feet of other existing shelters or other obstructions

Data from Refs. [2,5,13,34,51].

provide constant rather than intermittent airflow. In the winter, the goal of ventilation is to minimize airborne pathogen density, remove excess moisture from animal respiration, and maintain adequate ambient temperature (10–13°C, 50–55°F). Although higher ventilation rates improve air quality, they are inefficient because they require excessive heating costs. Supplemental heating may be necessary as the outside temperature falls or stocking density decreases. At optimal stocking densities, livestock generally produce enough animal heat to maintain adequate ambient temperature in confined housing when outside temperatures remain above −8°C [51]. Winter ventilation is a compromise between the removal of airborne contaminants and the maintenance of ambient temperature. The primary goal of summer ventilation is to minimize ambient temperature and relative humidity. This requires high ventilation flow rates, which also enhance air quality. The goal is to maintain an ambient housing temperature to no more than 2°C above the outside temperature [5,51].

Relative humidity levels should be maintained between 50% and 80%, and ammonia levels should not exceed 10 ppm [2,34,47,51,58]. Maximum recommended stocking densities should not be exceeded (see Table 2) [26]. Separate age groups of cattle should be maintained in separate barns or be separated by barrier walls. Calf hutches for individual dairy calves provide an ideal means of managing relative calf isolation and limiting airborne transmission if they are properly positioned and spaced. Recommendations for calf hutches include one calf per hutch with a minimum separation of 4 feet between hutches. Hutches should be placed at least 10 feet from older-cattle enclosures and 50 feet from livestock building exhaust fans.

Commingling and animal contact

Many cattle management systems provide numerous opportunities for exchange of respiratory pathogens from animal to animal. Assembling groups of beef calves for a feedlot often involves mixing calves from different origins, congregation of animals at sale barns or other holding pens, and movement in congested cattle transports. These activities are well known to increase the rate of respiratory disease occurrence by stressing the animals and providing circumstances that decrease disease resistance. These same animal contact and crowding circumstances can dramatically increase exposure to pathogens, often including pathogens to which the animal has not developed prior immunity.

In a recent national survey, more than 50% of dairy producers housed sick animals in a manner that allowed direct nose-to-nose contact with healthy herdmates [54]. Many dairy producers expand their herds by purchasing animals from other sources, but less than 25% of them provide any quarantine time for the incoming animals. For producers who introduced 15% or more of their total animal inventory during an expansion, 16.6% reported an increase in occurrence of respiratory disease during the year [55].

During the early phases of respiratory disease, the shedding rates of pathogens via respiratory secretions increases dramatically. Commingling, crowding, and the animal stresses that are involved in animal movement can precipitate respiratory problems. These same factors can increase spread of pathogens to other animals with close contact. Although quarantine may not be effective against diseases with chronic carrier states such as Johne's disease, it can substantially decrease the risk of spreading respiratory pathogens. Furthermore, the duration of respiratory pathogen shedding has also been well characterized. In general, nasal shedding of viral respiratory pathogens is significantly reduced by 14 days after infection but may persist longer in individual animals, which suggests that quarantine for approximately 14 to 21 days should significantly reduce the exposure and transmission of these pathogens within an operation. Practical suggestions for limiting pathogen spread by contact include quarantine of incoming livestock, maintenance of hospital areas that do not allow contact with healthy animals, prevention of animal contact between different age groups of cattle, minimizing the time animals spend in market channels, and limiting the introduction of new animals to assembled herds or pens of cattle.

The concepts of pathogen transmission within grouped housing can be effectively applied to weaned dairy calves. Calves receive relatively low pathogen exposure while in calf hutches. On weaning and grouping in calf pens, the risk of exposure increases dramatically. It is important to appreciate that the risk of exposure rises with the number of calves housed together. For example, if one estimates that 5% of calves born in a herd with bovine viral diarrhea virus are persistently infected, then the probability of bovine viral diarrhea virus exposure in a group of 10 calves is approximately 0.4 ($1-0.95^{10}$). If the stocking rate increases to 30 calves, the probability nearly doubles to 0.78 ($1-0.95^{30}$). Limiting the number of calves per pen to less than seven is associated with decreased respiratory disease mortality [28] (also see article by Smith in this issue).

It must be emphasized that one animal can expose an entire pen of animals by simple close contact, airborne transmission, or environmental transmission at common housing areas such as feed bunks and water troughs. By dividing animals into smaller groups, the number of animals exposed is lowered significantly. Using the same example of bovine viral diarrhea virus exposure, if one splits the 30 calves into three separate pens, the probability of having all 30 calves exposed to bovine viral diarrhea virus falls from 0.78 to the comparatively negligible level of 0.064 [$(1-0.95^{10})^3$]. Simple segregation of animals is not sufficient unless physical barriers for fence line contact, separation of food and water troughs, segregation of likely fomites, and blocking airborne spread are used. These same principles can be applied to any group-housing situation. Such management and housing decisions must be made based on a balance between the risk and cost of disease versus the availability and cost of facilities and labor.

*Minimizing the role of bovine viral diarrhea virus
in bovine respiratory disease*

It was noted previously that the common bovine respiratory pathogens are considered to be ubiquitous in cattle populations in the United States and most other countries. Although this does not suggest that every animal harbors each pathogen, these agents can be found routinely in the nasopharynx of healthy and diseased animals within most herds. In contrast, some European countries have successfully eradicated some viral respiratory pathogens such as bovine herpesvirus 1 and bovine viral diarrhea virus (BVDV) from cattle populations. Under the currently prevailing practices within the United States and many other countries, the authors do not suggest testing or identification of most respiratory pathogens as a viable means to identify carriers or to exclude the animals from introduction into a herd. The exception to this is BVDV. Although BVDV is not considered a primary pneumopathogen, it is considered to have an important role in respiratory disease of cattle [2,41]. The immunosuppressive effects of the virus and the close association of BVDV infection and respiratory disease occurrence in some epidemiologic studies suggest that the virus plays a role by promoting secondary bacterial lung infection.

Although BVDV vaccines have been improved over the past several years, vaccination alone rarely eliminates BVDV from an infected herd. An effective BVDV biosecurity program must include the identification and removal of persistently infected animals, BVDV screening of incoming animals and their calves, and a comprehensive vaccination program [7,8,25,57]. Persistently infected cattle do not mount an effective immune response against the virus and are capable of shedding large amounts of the virus into the environment through multiple routes. Persistently infected animals have been implicated as the primary means by which BVDV infection is maintained in assembled dairy herds, and they are also considered a significant threat for transmission in cow–calf and feedlot operations [20–23,32,50,60]. With the development of new tests over the past several years, our ability to accurately and expediently identify persistently infected animals has dramatically improved [9,25]. The serum immunoperoxidase monolayer assay (IPMA) and antigen capture ELISA tests and the immunohistochemistry test of skin biopsy material have appropriate sensitivity and specificity for detecting persistently infected cattle.

The authors do not know of significant published research that evaluates the effect of test-and-cull strategies for BVDV on the occurrence of BRDC; however, elimination of persistently infected animals from herds can have significant positive effects in decreasing other BVDV manifestations such as reproductive failure. Implementing test-and-cull procedures for persistently infected animals may prove to be a powerful means of decreasing BRDC prevalence.

In general, all cattle introduced into a herd should be tested for BVDV before purchase or entry. Acute BVDV infections of pregnant cattle can result in animals that are BVDV negative at the time of testing while the fetus is persistently infected. It is critical that all calves from newly introduced pregnant animals also be tested immediately after birth. To establish a BVDV-negative herd, it is generally more effective and economical to test calves as they are born rather than screen adult populations. A negative result for a calf indicates that not only the calf but also all of the calf's maternal ancestors are not persistently infected. A single positive test on a calf does not differentiate between acute and persistent infection. A confirmatory test may be performed in 4 weeks, or the animal may be assumed to be persistently infected and euthanized or sold for slaughter. The dams of all persistently infected calves should be traced and tested as well to determine their status. In most cases, these animals will test negative, indicating fetal exposure due to acute infection during gestation. Bulls should also be tested because they can contribute to animal exposure within a herd.

Summary

Although biosecurity practices play a role in minimizing respiratory disease in cattle, they must be used in combination with other management strategies that address the many other risk factors. Because the pathogens involved in bovine respiratory disease are enzootic in the general cattle population, biosecurity practices aimed at the complete elimination of exposure are currently impractical. Several animal husbandry and production management practices can be used to minimize pathogen shedding, exposure, and transmission within a given population, however. Various combinations of these control measures can be applied to individual farms to help decrease the morbidity and mortality attributed to respiratory disease.

References

[1] Ames TR. Dairy calf pneumonia: the disease and its impact. Vet Clin North Am Food Anim Pract 1997;13:379–91.

[2] Ames TR, Baker JC, Wikse SE. The bronchopneumonias (respiratory disease complex of cattle, sheep, and goats). In: Smith BP, editor. Large animal internal medicine, 3rd edition. St. Louis: Mosby; 2002. p. 551–70.

[3] Anderson JF, Bates DW. Appraising the adequacy of environment for confined animals. Vet Med Small Anim Clin 1979;74:208–10.

[4] Anderson JF, Bates DW. Influence of improved ventilation on health of confined cattle. J Am Vet Med Assoc 1979;174:577–80.

[5] Bates DW, Anderson JF. Calculation of ventilation needs for confined cattle. J Am Vet Med Assoc 1979;174:581–9.

[6] Beer M, Hehnen HR, Wolfmeyer A, et al. A new inactivated BVDV genotype I and II vaccine: an immunisation and challenge study with BVDV genotype I. Vet Microbiol 2000;77:195–208.

[7] Bitsch V, Ronsholt L. Control of bovine viral diarrhea virus infection without vaccines. Vet Clin North Am Food Anim Pract 1995;11:627–40.

[8] Bolin SR. Control of bovine viral diarrhea infection by use of vaccination. Vet Clin North Am Food Anim Pract 1995;11:615–25.

[9] Brock KV. Diagnosis of bovine viral diarrhea virus infections. Vet Clin North Am Food Anim Pract 1995;11:549–61.

[10] Christensen LS, Mortensen S, Botner A, et al. Further evidence of long distance airborne transmission of Aujeszky's disease (pseudorabies) virus. Vet Rec 1993;132:317–21.

[11] Christensen LS, Mousing J, Mortensen S, et al. Evidence of long distance airborne transmission of Aujeszky's disease (pseudorabies) virus. Vet Rec 1990;127:471–4.

[12] Cole NA. Preconditioning calves for the feedlot. Vet Clin North Am Food Anim Pract 1985;1:401–11.

[13] Collins Jr. ER. Ventilation of sheep and goat barns. Vet Clin North Am Food Anim Pract 1990;6:635–54.

[14] Curtis SE. Air environment and animal performance. J Anim Sci 1972;35:628–34.

[15] Daggupaty SM, Sellers RF. Airborne spread of foot-and-mouth disease in Saskatchewan. Canada, 1951–1952. Can J Vet Res 1990;54:465–8.

[16] Dean HJ, Leyh R. Cross-protective efficacy of a bovine viral diarrhea virus (BVDV) type 1 vaccine against BVDV type 2 challenge. Vaccine 1999;17:1117–24.

[17] Diesel DA, Lebel JL, Tucker A. Pulmonary particle deposition and airway mucociliary clearance in cold-exposed calves. Am J Vet Res 1991;52:1665–71.

[18] Donaldson AI. Factors influencing the dispersal, survival and deposition of airborne pathogens of farm animals. Vet Bull 1978;48:83–94.

[19] Hillman P, Gebremedhin K, Warner R. Ventilation system to minimize airborne bacteria, dust, humidity, and ammonia in calf nurseries. J Dairy Sci 1992;75:1305–12.

[20] Houe H. Age distribution of animals persistently infected with bovine virus diarrhea virus in twenty-two Danish dairy herds. Can J Vet Res 1992;56:194–8.

[21] Houe H. Epidemiological features and economical importance of bovine virus diarrhoea virus (BVDV) infections. Vet Microbiol 1999;64:89–107.

[22] Houe H. Epidemiology of bovine viral diarrhea virus. Vet Clin North Am Food Anim Pract 1995;11:521–47.

[23] Houe H, Baker JC, Maes RK, et al. Prevalence of cattle persistently infected with bovine viral diarrhea virus in 20 dairy herds in two counties in central Michigan and comparison of prevalence of antibody-positive cattle among herds with different infection and vaccination status. J Vet Diagn Invest 1995;7:321–6.

[24] Hum S, Kessell A, Djordjevic S, et al. Mastitis, polyarthritis and abortion caused by Mycoplasma species bovine group 7 in dairy cattle. Aust Vet J 2000;78:744–50.

[25] Kelling CL, Grotelueschen DM, Smith DR, et al. Testing and management strategies for effective beef and dairy herd BVDV biosecurity programs. The Bovine Practitioner 2000;34: 13–22.

[26] Klingborg DJ. Preventing calf pneumonia. Compend Contin Educ Pract Vet 1986;8: F112–4.

[27] Linklater KA, Watson GA. Sheep housing and health. Vet Rec 1983;113:560–4.

[28] Losinger WC, Heinrichs AJ. Management variables associated with high mortality rates attributable to respiratory tract problems in female calves prior to weaning. J Am Vet Med Assoc 1996;209:1756–9.

[29] Mars MH, Bruschke CJ, van Oirschot JT. Airborne transmission of BHV1. BRSV, and BVDV among cattle is possible under experimental conditions. Vet Microbiol 1999;66: 197–207.

[30] Mars MH, de Jong MC, van Maanen C, et al. Airborne transmission of bovine herpesvirus 1 infections in calves under field conditions. Vet Microbiol 2000;76:1–3.

[31] Meyer VM. Ventilation systems for swine housing. Vet Med Small Anim Clin 1975;70: 992–3.

[32] Moerman A, Straver PJ, de Jong MC, et al. A long term epidemiological study of bovine viral diarrhoea infections in a large herd of dairy cattle. Vet Rec 1993;132:622–6.

[33] Nardell EA, Keegan J, Cheney SA, et al. Airborne infection: Theoretical limits of protection achievable by building ventilation. Am Rev Respir Dis 1991;144:302–6.

[34] Parker WH. Housing of ruminants: II. requirements of good housing and effects of bad housing. Vet Rec 1968;83:364–8.

[35] Perino LJ. Advances in pulmonary immunology. Vet Clin North Am Food Anim Pract 1997;13:393–9.

[36] Perino, LJ, Wittum, TE, Ross, GS, et al. Failure of passive transfer: risk factors and effects on lifetime performance. In: Proceedings of the American Association of Bovine Practitioners, 28th Annual AABP Convention. San Antonio (TX); 1996. p. 101–10.

[37] Pfutzner H, Sachse K. *Mycoplasma bovis* as an agent of mastitis, pneumonia, arthritis and genital disorders in cattle. Rev Sci Tech 1996;15:1477–94.

[38] Pickrell J. Hazards in confinement housing—gases and dusts in confined animal houses for swine, poultry, horses and humans. Vet Hum Toxicol 1991;33:32–9.

[39] Pickrell JA, Heber AJ, Murphy JP, et al. Characterization of particles, ammonia and endotoxin in swine confinement operations. Vet Hum Toxicol 1993;35:421–8.

[40] Pierson RE, Kainer RA. Clinical classification of pneumonias in cattle. The Bovine Practitioner 1980;15:73–9.

[41] Potgieter LN. Bovine respiratory tract disease caused by bovine viral diarrhea virus. Vet Clin North Am Food Anim Pract 1997;13:471–81.

[42] Ribble CS. Assessing vaccine efficacy. Can Vet J 1990;31:679–81.

[43] Sainsbury DW. Housing of livestock: II. practical considerations of ventilation and construction. Veterinarian 1966;4:29–32.

[44] Sivula NJ, Ames TR, Marsh WE, et al. Descriptive epidemiology of morbidity and mortality in Minnesota dairy heifer calves. Prev Vet Med 1996;27:155–71.

[45] Sorensen JH, Mackay DK, Jensen CO, et al. An integrated model to predict the atmospheric spread of foot-and-mouth disease virus. Epidemiol Infect 2000;124:577–90.

[46] Speer NC, Young C, Roeber D. The importance of preventing bovine respiratory disease: A beef industry review. The Bovine Practitioner 2001;35:189–96.

[47] Stark KD. The role of infectious aerosols in disease transmission in pigs. Vet J 1999;158:164–81.

[48] Step DL. Mycoplasma infection in cattle: I pneumonia-arthritis syndrome. The Bovine Practitioner 2001;35:149–55.

[49] Stipkovits L, Ripley P, Varga J, et al. Clinical study of the disease of calves associated with *Mycoplasma bovis* infection. Acta Vet Hung 2000;48:387–95.

[50] Taylor LF, Van Donkersgoed J, Dubovi EJ, et al. The prevalence of bovine viral diarrhea virus infection in a population of feedlot calves in western Canada. Can J Vet Res 1995;59:87–93.

[51] Turnbull JE. Housing and environment for dairy calves. Can Vet J 1980;21:85–90.

[52] USDA. APHIS:VS Centers for Epidemiology and Animal Health NAHMS. Beef '97, part II: reference of 1997 beef cow-calf health & health management practices, 1997, Report #N238.797.

[53] USDA. APHIS:VS Centers for Epidemiology and Animal Health NAHMS. Cattle and calves death loss, 1995, Report #N232.397.

[54] USDA. APHIS:VS Centers for Epidemiology and Animal Health NAHMS. Dairy '96, part I: reference of 1996 dairy management practices, 1996, Report #N200.696.

[55] USDA. APHIS:VS Centers for Epidemiology and Animal Health NAHMS. Dairy '96, part III: reference of 1996 dairy health and health management, 1996, Report #N212.1196.

[56] USDA. APHIS:VS Centers for Epidemiology and Animal Health NAHMS. Feedlot '99, part III: health management and biosecurity in U.S. feedlots, 2000, Report #N336.1200.

[57] Van Oirschot JT, Bruschke CJ, van Rijn PA. Vaccination of cattle against bovine viral diarrhoea. Vet Microbiol 1999;64:169–83.

[58] Wathes CM, Jones CD, Webster AJ. Ventilation, air hygiene and animal health. Vet Rec 1983;113:554–9.
[59] West K, Petrie L, Konoby C, et al. The efficacy of modified-live bovine respiratory syncytial virus vaccines in experimentally infected calves. Vaccine 1999;18:907–19.
[60] Wittum TE, Grotelueschen DM, Brock KV, et al. Persistent bovine viral diarrhoea virus infection in US beef herds. Prev Vet Med 2001;49:83–94.

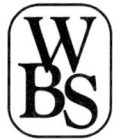

THE VETERINARY
CLINICS
Food Animal
Practice

Vet Clin Food Anim 18 (2002) 79–98

Biosecurity for reproductive diseases

Michael W. Sanderson, DVM, MS[a],*, David P. Gnad, DVM[b]

[a]Department of Clinical Sciences, 111B Mosier Hall,
Kansas State University, Manhattan, KS 66506-5706 USA
[b]Veterinary Medical Teaching Hospital, 106A Mosier Hall, Kansas State University,
Manhattan, KS 66506-5701 USA

Optimal reproductive performance is key for beef and dairy breeding herds and reproductive disease can have a major effect on reproductive efficiency of a herd. Identification of reproductive pathogens however, can be challenging. Only 23–46% of abortions submitted to a diagnostic laboratory are diagnosed with a specific cause [9]. In beef herds, infertility is often not recognized until 3–5 months after breeding when cows are examined for pregnancy. This time lag complicates identification of reproductive pathogens. As with all diseases, diagnostic tests do not perform flawlessly and so need to be rationally applied and interpreted. For all these reasons, a proactive plan to protect the fertility of the herd is important. Producers are often uncertain on the proper application of biosecurity tools. Veterinarians with sufficient understanding of disease epidemiology, test and vaccine performance, and risk assessment can provide rational guidance on the proper development and implementation of a biosecurity plan. This plan will be based on the particular herd's current disease status, the specific disease to be controlled, cost of prevention, likelihood of an outbreak, impact of an outbreak, and risk aversion of the producer.

Multiple tools are available to decrease the risk of importing disease into a herd including implementing testing, quarantine, and vaccination requirements. Perhaps the most important tool is to only import cattle from herds with known health status. We then only import from disease free herds or herds with an appropriate vaccination program and records of excellent reproductive performance. Knowledge of the health status and performance of the whole herd of origin is more valuable than the results of tests on one or a few animals from the herd (see chapter 9 by Smith [88]).

* Corresponding author.
E-mail address: sandersn@vet.ksu.edu (M.W. Sanderson).

For the reproductive diseases of importance most herds become infected through the importation of an infected animal. Campylobacter and Trichomonas are venereal diseases so they only enter with an infected breeding age animal. IBR and BVD are ubiquitous agents and can enter the herd through the importation of any age animal including replacement calves, stockers, and breeding stock. BVD may have other reservoirs as well but they are not likely a common way for disease to enter a herd. Neospora and Leptospira may enter the herd through an imported, infected animal of any age class. They each also have an outside reservoir that may introduce disease to a herd even in the absence of imports, so control efforts must include management of the environment and reservoir. Understanding the epidemiology of various pathogens will allow the clinician to customize a biosecurity plan for the operation.

Leptospirosis

Importance

Leptospirosis is an important cause of abortion and infertility in North American cattle. The species of concern for veterinary medicine were previously all classified as *Leptospira interrogans* but have recently been reorganized into seven different species, each with multiple serovars. Over 200 serovars of *Leptospira* are recognized worldwide. Serovars of importance in cattle within *L. interrogans* include bratislava, canicola, icterohaemorrhagiae, and pomona. The newly defined species *Leptospira borgpetersenii* includes serovar *hardjo* and *Leptospira kirschneri* includes serovar *grippotyphosa*. In a survey of US slaughter cows, 2% were renal carriers and 49% had antibodies to Leptospira species [70]. Elevated titers to Leptospira have been associated with increased fetal loss in dairy cows [42,93]. Most renal isolates (83%) were identified as serovar *hardjo* but *pomona* (12.5%) and *grippotyphosa* (4.5%) were also found [70]. Renal isolation and seroprevalence were more common in the southeast, south central and pacific coast states than elsewhere in the US [71]. Leptospira species usually cause late term abortions in cattle. In one diagnostic lab survey over 10 years Leptospira species accounted for 6% of diagnosed bacterial causes of abortion. The most common bacteria isolated in the survey were opportunists, generally considered to be sporadic causes of abortion [52]. Leptospira species may also cause infertility in cattle. Recent research shows an increase in calving to conception interval and services per conception among cows with elevated titers to serovar hardjo [40]. A recent general review of Leptospirosis is available [15].

Reservoir and transmission

Methods of transmission and risks are dependent on whether the serovar involved is host adapted or incidental. Incidental serovars are adapted to and maintained in other species but may infect cattle. The host adapted serovar for cattle is *Leptospira borgpetersenii* serovar *hardjo*. Host adapted serovars generally cause less clinical disease in the adult and result in a longer period of shedding from the kidney and genital tract. Cattle serve as the maintenance host for serovar hardjo. Transmission may occur through contaminated environmental sources such as water or by venereal transmission. All other serovars result in incidental infection in cattle. The most common incidental serovars associated with abortion in cattle are *L. interrogans* serovar *pomona* and *Leptospira kirschneri* serovar *grippotyphosa*. Host adapted, maintenance species for these serovars include skunks, opossums, raccoons squirrels and swine. Environmental transmission of *L. interrogans* serovar *pomona* from pigs to cattle in mixed farms can occur [41]. Other serovars may infect cattle as well and may include a broad range of maintenance hosts. Transmission of incidental infections is through contact with a contaminated environment. Environmental conditions suitable for survival of *Leptospira* species are important for transmission. Survival and thus exposure to Leptospires is facilitated in moderate temperatures, and standing water. Leptospires may invade through intact oral mucosa or water saturated skin. Environments with standing water provide a suitable environment for the bacteria as well as softening the skin of the coronary band to facilitate infection. Invading Leptospires are hemotogenously spread to the mammary gland, kidney, and reproductive tract. Once a cow is infected, Leptospires are shed from the affected organ for a variable period of time depending on the host adaptation of the serovar and the immune response of the animal. Risk of infection for cattle in a herd comes from persistently shedding cattle or from outside species. Cows that chronically shed serovar *hardjo* in their urine may spread the organism by contaminating the environment resulting in indirect spread or by direct venereal spread between cows and bulls. Infected bulls may shed Leptospires in semen and urine for months, contaminating the environment and potentially transmitting the infection during breeding. Cattle may also be indirectly exposed to Leptospires by environmental contamination from other species of domestic animals or wildlife. The herd is placed at risk or potentially exposed to Leptospires when a shedding cow is imported to the herd. Alternately, an increase in the population of wildlife may contaminate cattle holding pens. Coupled with environmental conditions that favor Leptospire survival, the risk for an outbreak increases. Knowledge of the specific serovar involved in an outbreak is useful in identifying proper biocontainment steps for control.

Transmission may be possible through embryo transfer as well. In experimental studies, Leptospires can be identified in uterine and oviductal fluids by culture and in cultured embryos by PCR [11]. Leptospires could not be isolated from oocytes exposed during in-vitro fertilization when cultured in the presence of streptomycin and penicillin. In contrast, when culture media did not contain antibiotics, sequential wash procedures did not remove all Leptospires [12]. Semen may also contain Leptospires and if not handled correctly can survive the freezing process and potentially be a source of infection. Proper monitoring of bulls for infection at the bull stud and appropriate semen preparation for freezing can minimize this risk. Semen should only be purchased from bull studs with adequate procedures in place to prevent Leptospira contamination of semen.

Prevention and control

Quarantine and testing

If 2% is an accurate estimate of the number of cows shedding *Leptospira* spp in their urine [70], importation of chronically shedding cattle is clearly a risk for introduction of Leptospirosis to a herd. Importation only from herds with records of excellent reproductive performance will decrease the risk of importing a shedding animal. Cattle infected with the serovar hardjo are typically normal clinically and continue to shed for months to years. Quarantine alone then is not effective in preventing introduction of this form of Leptospira. Quarantine could be effective in segregating imported animals until testing could determine their infection status. Runoff from the quarantine area must be controlled and not allowed to contact the resident herd. Tests available for detection of *Leptospira* ssp in imported cattle include serology and culture. Titers to hardjo in chronically shedding cattle are often <1:100 [50] so serology alone may fail to identify many cases. A positive serologic response to hardjo indicates recent infection but does not define the shedding status of the animal, a negative serologic titer is meaningless. Culture of urine for identification is definitive but Leptospires are difficult to grow in the lab so false negative cultures are a problem. Culture sensitivity may be as low as 17% in some situations although sensitivity of culture of non-vaccinated cows was better [17], presumably due to decreased shedding or antibody interference in vaccinated cows. A positive culture is definitive but a negative culture does not mean the animal is not shedding hardjo. The polymerase chain reaction (PCR) has been used in a research setting to identify Leptospires in bovine urine [68] and semen [43]. While highly sensitive, even minute amounts of contamination from positive samples can result in false positive reactions. In the final analysis, identification of cattle chronically infected with host adapted serovar hardjo is problematic. An alternative approach is to treat all imported cattle with antibiotics to clear any infection during a quarantine period. In a recent study, one dose of long acting oxytetracycline at 20mg/kg eliminated renal shedding of *Leptospira borgpetersenii* serovar hardjo in experimentally infected cattle [2]. Urine was negative for Leptospires by PCR, darkfield microscopy, immunofluorescence testing and microbial culture beginning 1 week after treatment through 6 weeks post treatment [2].

Vaccination

Vaccination of the resident herd and imported animals may be a useful way to provide some level of protection for the herd. Challenge trials involving currently available vaccines indicate they do not prevent colonization of the kidneys and shedding of Leptospires in the urine, or abortion in pregnant cattle [16,18]. Other studies however, suggest that fertility may be improved in herds that vaccinate for Leptospirosis through decreased days open and higher first service conception rate [33,40]. An experimental vaccine has been effective in controlling infection in a herd in Scotland along with quarantine and streptomycin treatment of all imported animals [60]. A vaccine available in Australia, New Zealand and the United Kingdom protected vaccinated heifers from renal colonization and urine shedding while control heifers showed renal colonization and urine shedding [14]. Required frequency of vaccination varies with the level of exposure. Herds in semi-arid regions often vaccinate one time per year with no apparent breaks in protection. In beef herds this is often done at the time of pregnancy examination in early to mid-gestation. In wetter environments with higher exposure, vaccination 2–3 times per year may be necessary to achieve control. Prebreeding and mid gestation vaccination may assist in control of both abortion and infertility.

Environmental control

Particularly in wetter climates, control of the environment may be important in reducing the exposure level of cows. Any steps that can decrease the environmental survival of Leptospires will decrease cow exposure. Increased population density of cows (i.e. corrals or small pasture) can increase environmental contamination levels so population density should be controlled as much as possible consistent with management needs and goals. Additionally, corrals should be graded to prevent standing water as areas of standing water provide a suitable environment for Leptospire survival. A mild slope to the corral and a relatively impervious surface will aid water drainage. Wildlife may also be a source of incidental infection for cattle and a program to limit contact between wildlife and cattle, pens, feed, and water may be helpful.

Trichomonas

Importance

Trichomonas foetus is a venereally transmitted protozoan parasite of the bovine. The primary reservoir is the persistently infected bull. Estimates of prevalence of *Trichomonas* in individual bulls surveyed at slaughter houses range from less than 1% [39] to 7% [56] and herd prevalence in farm surveys from 16% [19] to 44% [54]. A planned prevalence survey of 57 of 60 randomly selected cow-calf herds in California found 4% of bulls and 16% of herds positive for *Trichomonas* [19]. Simulation models of the impact of *Trichomonas* infection on cow calf profitability suggest a 5–35% decrease in revenue depending on the prevalence of infection among the bulls [79]. Rae et al found a prevalence of 11.9% among bulls in a large multi-unit ranch with the prevalence in individual units ranging from 0% to 35.9% [80]. A significant negative association was noted between unit bull prevalence and the weaning percent and weaning weight per exposed cow for that unit [80]. Initial conception rates are normal in the face of *Trichomonas* infection but decrease markedly by 90–120 days of gestation. *Trichomonas* infection results in depressed pregnancy rates in acute [55] and endemically infected herds [89].

Reservoir and transmission

Trichomonas foetus is a venereally transmitted disease and the bull is the primary reservoir. Importation of non-virgin cattle into the herd or allowing contact with other herds increases risk for trichomonas introduction. Bulls usually become colonized after breeding an infected cow, and carry the organism in the crypts of the glans penis and the fornix of the prepuce. As bulls age they are more likely to become persistently colonized after exposure apparently due to deepening of the mucosal crypts of the penis and prepuce producing a more favorable microenvironment for trichomonad survival. In a survey of bulls in California 0.5% of bulls 2 years old or younger were positive (1/221), while 6.2% of bulls 3years old and older were positive (29/465) [19]. Although young bulls only occasionally become persistently infected they can certainly serve as mechanical transmitters after breeding an infected cow. The only bulls that can be certain of not being infected are true virgin bulls. Reports of infection in virgin bulls appear to be due to a different trichomonad that may be a contaminant from feces [20]. Cows typically clear infection after several heat cycles. Approximately 1% of infected cows may remain persistently infected after abortion and up to 5% of cows can maintain infection through gestation and into the post partum period [87], potentially serving as a source of infection to the herd. Communal grazing is a risk for herd infection as well. In Idaho herds that practiced communal grazing, an increasing number of herds grazing together was associated with increased risk for herd infection [38].

Prevention and control

Quarantine and testing

Importation only from herds with records of excellent reproductive performance will decrease the risk of importing an infected animal. The only animals that pose no risk to the herd from *Trichomonas* are true virgin animals. If there is any doubt as to the status of an animal, testing is advisable. Quarantine alone will not be effective in excluding *Trichomonas* from a herd since persistently colonized bulls show no clinical signs. A quarantine period to allow for testing of imports before their entry into the herd can however be effective. The standard testing method is to scrape the mucosa of the penis and prepuce with an insemination pipette while aspirating with a 20cc syringe. The collected smega is inoculated into Diamonds media or a commercially available media (InPouch TF, BioMed Diagnostics, San Jose, CA). The commercially available media has an extended shelf life and may serve as culture media or transport media to a diagnostic lab. The sensitivity of the collection technique and incubation in commercial media has been estimated at 70% [80] to 97% [56]. For the individual bull in quarantine prior to joining the herd, 3 consecutive negative tests should be performed to assure the bull is not infected. Sexual activity is thought to decrease the number of trichomonads in the prepuce, thereby decreasing test sensitivity so testing should begin after a period of sexual rest. Importing cows to the herd entails risk as well. Chronically infected cows may serve as a source of infection for the herd. If a reproductive exam or the reproductive history of the imported cows is suspicious, they should similarly be quarantined and tested by culturing cervical mucus prior to entry to the herd. Ideally, mature cows should only be imported from herds where the reproductive performance of the herd is known to be acceptable.

Samples inoculated into the commercial media (InPouch TF, BioMed Diagnostics, San Jose, CA) may be incubated at the clinic and read at 1, 2, 3 and 7 days using 100X magnification. Trichomonads may be recognized by their characteristic motility and morphology. A morphologically similar trichomonad has been identified that is thought to be a commensal inhabitant of the lower bowel. False positive cultures have been reported potentially arising from fecal contamination of the sample [20]. If this is suspected, the species can be differentiated by PCR [20]. Care should be taken when obtaining samples to avoid fecal contamination, including cleaning of the external prepuce if necessary.

Vaccination

Vaccines are available for *Trichomonas*, alone or in combination with *Campylobacter* and *Leptospira* antigens. Vaccination may be a useful adjunct to good management practices to decrease the risk from *Trichomonas*. It will not however, prevent infection and reproductive losses. Vaccine trials suggest the vaccine is effective in decreasing the duration of shedding, and increasing pregnancy rates following exposure [54,55]. In one study 62.5% of challenged vaccinated heifers produced calves versus 31.5% of challenged control heifers produced calves (vaccine efficacy 45%) [55]. As such it may be an effective measure in the face of an outbreak to decrease losses while management efforts work to eradicate the infection from the herd.

Herd management

A review of control methods for *Trichomonas* is available [56]. Briefly, *Trichomonas* can be kept out by importing only true virgin animals to the herd or quarantine and serial testing of non-virgin animals. Communal grazing during periods of sexual activity increase risk and should be avoided if possible. Alternately, producer groups may initiate collective monitoring or eradication efforts to control risk. Once *Trichomonas* is introduced into a herd, eradication will require additional efforts. All bulls should be serially cultured and infected bulls must be culled from the herd. Carrier cows may also serve as a source of infection for the herd. Open and late calving cows should be culled to decrease the risk from carrier cows [56]. Artificial insemination can be an effective management tool in the control of *Trichomonas*. Semen should be acquired from bull studs with testing protocols for *Trichomonas* [72].

Campylobacteriosis

Importance

Campylobacter fetus subspecies *venerealis* is a venereally transmitted disease in the bovine. Prevalence of infection in North America is unknown but clinical disease seems rare. The widespread use of artificial insemination using semen from reputable bull studs has minimized the occurrence in dairy herds. Occasional outbreaks occur due to breaks in management. Introduction of *Campylobacter fetus* subspecies *venerealis* into a herd may cause marked infertility and early embryonic death. Initially, pregnancy rates are markedly decreased across cow ages followed by lower level infertility in cows as they build immunity and marked infertility in naive heifers. Along with *Leptospira*, *Campylobacter* is the most common vaccine given to cows [81,82].

Reservoir and transmission

The primary reservoir for *Campylobacter* is the persistently infected bull. Colonization occurs in the crypts of the glans penis and prepuce of the bull. Older bulls are persistently infected more commonly than young bulls. The persistently colonized bull transmits infection to cows during service and transiently colonized bulls can serve as a mechanical transmitter. Additionally, bulls can become infected from contaminated bedding used previously by infected bulls [32]. Cows generally clear infection within 3–6 months however they may rarely harbor the organism in the reproductive tract for over a year [101].

Prevention and control

Quarantine and testing

Importation of colonized bulls or infected cows is the main route of introduction to the herd. Exposure to neighbor's bulls through communal grazing or fence breaks may also serve as a source of exposure. Importation only from herds with records of excellent reproductive performance will decrease the risk of importing an infected animal. Quarantine and testing of all non-virgin bulls prior to contact with the herd can effectively prevent introduction of colonized bulls. As for Trichomonas, if a reproductive exam or the reproductive history of the imported cows are suspicious, they should be quarantined and tested by culturing cervical mucus prior to entry to the herd. Ideally, mature cows should only be imported from herds where the reproductive performance of the herd is known to be acceptable.

Campylobacter is difficult to culture and specific transport media should be used to optimize sensitivity of culture [49]. Contact your local diagnostic lab for transport recommendations. Serial cultures should be taken at 1 week intervals for 3 weeks to increase the likelihood that infected bulls will be identified.

Vaccination

Vaccines for *Campylobacter* are available either alone or in combination with *Leptospira*. Field trial data suggest that *Campylobacter* vaccination is effective in decreasing the effect of disease on the herd. Vaccine efficacy in multiple field trials ranged from 38% to 67% in cows [1,27,45]. Vaccination appears to be more effective when given close to the time of breeding compared to earlier. Heifers given their booster vaccination 4½ months prior to breeding had a pregnancy rate of 54% following a 63 day breeding season versus 92% in heifers given their booster vaccination 10 days prior to breeding [10]. In bulls, vaccination also provides protection from persistent colonization [25,26,36]. In one study vaccinated bulls did not become persistently colonized after breeding infected heifers but non-vaccinated bulls did become persistently colonized. Vaccinated bulls were however, able to mechanically transmit disease [36]. Vaccination may also be useful for treating colonized animals. In naturally colonized bulls, Bouters et al reported clearance rates of 70% of 41 bulls following one vaccination and 100% after a second vaccination 6 weeks later, however there were no control animals [21]. In experimentally colonized bulls, 6 of 6 bulls were culture negative by 4 weeks after a second vaccination and did not infect heifers they were bred to, while 4 of 4 control bulls remained culture positive and did infect heifers they were bred to [98]. Vaccination may not be effective in all bulls however [48]. Vaccination increased cure rates in experimentally colonized heifers compared to non-vaccinated controls as well [86]. Vaccination should not be relied upon to clear colonization in bulls or cows without multiple follow-up cultures to assure that clearance has taken place.

Bovine viral diarrhea

Importance

Bovine viral diarrhea virus (BVDV) is a common infection of cattle around the world. Surveys show individual seroprevalence of 65–75%, prevalence of persistent infection (PI) of 2%, and herd seroprevalence of 80–100% [46]. BVDV infection may cause decreased fertility [66], abortions, birth of congenitally abnormal calves, and the birth of persistently infected calves that may perform poorly and typically die by 1 year of age. In a 10 year diagnostic lab survey of causes of abortion, 4.5% of all abortions submitted were attributed to BVDV. Of abortions attributed to viral causes 43% were attributed to BVDV [51].

Reservoir and transmission

Bovine Viral Diarrhea Virus is predominantly spread from animal to animal by direct nose to nose contact. Any method of transfer of infective secretions may transmit infection however, including semen [53], contaminated needles, aerosols [62], biting flies [90], and rectal palpation [57]. The primary source of infection in an endemic herd is the persistently infected animal [46]. These animals shed high numbers of viral particles. Acute infections likely also play a role in the maintenance of infection in the herd but acutely infected animals shed fewer virus particles and for a much shorter period of time. Importation of a new animal, persistently or acutely infected, to the herd frequently precedes an outbreak of BVD. Exposure of pregnant cows or heifers to BVDV from this imported animal from 45–125 days of gestation may result in persistently infected calves that expose the rest of the herd well after the initial outbreak. Contact with neighboring cattle herds also provides some risk to the resident herd. Additional outside reservoirs may exist in sheep [23], swine and wildlife [61,73]. Infection of some wild ruminants with BVDV is possible [91], but the incidence of adequate contact resulting in transmission is unknown. Some serologic evidence of BVDV infection in wild ruminants may be more related to a different pestivirus with serological cross reactivity rather than actual BVDV infection. The importance of non-bovine hosts in the epidemiology of BVDV in the cattle population is not clear. An excellent review of the epidemiology of BVDV is available [46].

Prevention and control

Quarantine and testing

Preventing BVDV from entering a herd revolves around identification of acute and persistent infections in imported animals prior to introduction into the herd. Ideally, imports should only come from herds with records of excellent general health and reproductive performance to decrease the risk of importing a positive animal. Recent advances in diagnostic testing for BVDV have improved our ability to identify and exclude infected animals. Quarantine, while effective for limiting exposure to acutely ill animals, is not adequate to exclude BVDV from a herd since persistently infected animals may appear normal and not manifest disease during a quarantine period. Diagnostic testing is necessary in conjunction with quarantine during the time that tests are pending. Virus isolation from blood has been the standard test to identify animals with viremia. Persistently infected animals will have high levels of virus in blood and the viremia will persist over time. Two positive samples separated by 3 weeks are definitive for persistent infection. If a persistently infected animal is identified during quarantine it should be immediately culled. Acutely infected animals will not remain viremic. Acute infections will resolve and the animal will be safe to add to the herd.

Once a herd has a BVDV infection, control within the herd is more challenging. As the persistently infected animal is the main source of continuing infection for the herd, their identification and removal is critical. Identification of PI animals may require testing of the whole herd initially. Most PI animals die by 1 year of age, however some may survive and produce for a number of years. Alternately, all calves can be tested for virus and the dams of any positive calves tested. Ideally, PI calves and cows should be identified and removed prior to the onset of the breeding season to prevent exposure of cows in early to mid gestation. Two tests have recently become available that facilitate testing of whole herds. Virus isolation in 96 well microtitre plates followed by detection with ELISA [84,85], and imunohistochemistry of ear notch skin biopsies [85,92] have proven to be economical and practical for use at the herd level. Skin biopsy immunohistochemistry may be useful in differentiating acute infections from persistent infection, however additional data are needed to confirm this observation [74]. Individuals positive on virus isolation should be retested 3 weeks after the initial sampling to differentiate acute and persistent infections. Maternally derived antibody can interfere with isolation of the virus from blood early in life. Use of whole blood and isolation from white blood cell lysates can overcome this problem. Testing of all calves after maternal antibody levels have fallen (4–6 months of age) can be effective. Serology on unvaccinated calves at 6–7 months of age may effectively identify herds with a persistently infected individual [47]. The presence of positive titers in this unvaccinated group indicates exposure to a persistently infected individual and indicates further testing is needed.

Vaccination

Vaccination can be a useful adjunct to proper management in the control of reproductive disease from BVDV. The vaccination must provide fetal protection in order to be useful in a control program. Available evidence suggests that vaccination may provide some level of fetal protection. In one study utilizing an inactivated vaccine, 5 of 5 non-vaccinated heifers delivered persistently infected calves while only 3 of 7 vaccinated heifers produced PI calves [69]. In a recent study involving modified live virus vaccine, 6 unvaccinated controls and 12 vaccinates were challenged and pregnancies followed to term. All calves born to control heifers were persistently infected (6/6). Among the vaccinates, 2 of 11 calves born to heifers that delivered full term calves were persistently infected. One heifer aborted at 200 days gestation but no BVDV was found [28]. Clearly this level of protection will not prevent the birth of persistently infected calves if biosecurity methods allow introduction of infected cattle. It will however limit the effect of an inadvertent introduction of BVDV whether from imported cattle, contact with neighboring cattle or an outside reservoir.

Infectious bovine rhinotracheitis

Importance

Bovine Herpes Virus 1 is the causative agent of Infectious Bovine Rhinotracheitis (IBR) causing both infertility and abortion in cattle. Seroprevalence studies suggest that BHV-1 infection is widely distributed in cattle herds [102]. In susceptible herds 25–60% of cows may abort following exposure during pregnancy. Infertility or early embryonic death may result from necrotizing endometritis or oophoritis following infection around the time of breeding. In a 10 year diagnostic lab survey of causes of abortion, IBR was detected in 5.4% of all abortions submitted and 51% of abortions attributed to viral causes [51].

Reservoir and transmission

Bovine Herpes virus causes a latent infection in cattle, residing in the trigeminal and sacral ganglia [75]. These latent infections may be reactivated by stressful conditions. Because of this reactivation, cattle previously exposed to BHV-1 can serve as a source of infection for susceptible animals [8]. Persistence of infection in the herd is a result of both acute infections in susceptible animals and reactivation of shedding in latently infected animals.

Prevention and control

Quarantine and testing

A period of quarantine to allow possible acute or reactivated infections to manifest and resolve may be useful to avoid introducing active infection. Any seropositive animal may serve as a source of infection to a negative herd when reactivation of shedding occurs. Exclusion of seropositive animals without establishing a negative herd is of no value. If a negative herd is to be established, strict import, quarantine and testing requirements must be instituted to prevent reintroduction of virus to the herd.

Vaccination

Vaccination is commonly used as a preventative for disease among herds that utilize veterinary services [81], but less so in randomly selected herds [82]. Both modified live virus and killed products are available. Vaccine efficacy in an experimental study involving a modified live virus vaccine was 90% 7 months after vaccination, 1 of 10 vaccinated heifers aborted and 10 of 10 control heifers aborted [29]. Vaccination will not prevent establishment of latency and modified live virus vaccination may induce latency.

Neosporosis

Importance

Neospora caninum has become a commonly recognized cause of bovine abortion in California dairy cattle [3] and in beef cattle [44,99,100]. It has also been associated with increased culling [94] and decreased milk production [95]. Evidence of *Neospora* infection is common in U.S. beef and dairy herds. Overall herd seroprevalence in a 55 herd seroprevalence survey was 23% with individual within herd seroprevalence ranging from 2.5% to 67% [83]. Other studies have shown similar seroprevalence in beef herds [78,99]. A prevalence survey in Spain found an overall seroprevalence of 18% in 216 beef herds but with 97 (45%) having no seropositive animals [78]. In dairy surveys, overall animal prevalence has been approximately 17% with a range of 0 to 55% [30,77].

Reservoir and transmission

Neospora caninum is an apicomplexa protozoan, morphologically similar to *Toxoplasma gondii* and *Sarcocystis* species. The life cycle of *N. caninum*, and the associated risk factors for bovine infection have not been completely defined. Vertical transmission [13,31,76] has been shown to be common, approximately 92% of dams transmit infection to their fetuses [31]. Colostrum inoculated with *Neospora* tachyzoites has also been shown to transmit infection experimentally [97], but shedding of *Neospora* tachyzoites in milk has not been shown. Available evidence indicates horizontal transmission also occurs [65]. Recent studies show that dogs are a definitive host for *N. caninum* [58,64] and widespread seropositivity has been established in domestic and wild canids [6,22,59]. A number of species appear to be able to serve as intermediate hosts including deer [35] and domestic pigeons

[67], and may serve as a source of infection for dogs and wild canids. Inges-tion of oocysts from the feces of a definitive host such as dogs or wild canids has been hypothesized as a route of horizontal transmission [63]. Increased seroprevalence on ranches has been associated with increased cow density [7,83] and with increased wild canid density [7]. Seropositive cows com-monly transmit infection to their offspring, and tissues from abortions may infect canines [34] each serving to maintain infection in a herd. Serostatus of the individual cow has been associated with abortion risk [99] but not been consistently associated with pregnancy status [83,99]. Timing of infection or recrudescence may be important in determining the outcome of *Neospora* infection [103].

Prevention and control

Quarantine and testing

A multitude of diagnostic tests to identify a serologic response to *Neos-pora caninum* have been reported in the literature. An ELISA test kit is commercially available (HerdChek®, IDEXX, Westbrook, MA). Ideally, im-ports should only come from herds with records of excellent reproductive performance to decrease the risk of importing a problem animal. Seroposi-tive cows are not a risk to the herd until calving when an infected calf may be born or a canine infected by placental tissues. Seropositive cows are how-ever, more likely to abort [96,104]. Mathematical modeling of *Neospora* infection in dairy herds suggests that culling seropositive cattle is an effective method of control. Prevalence did not reach zero in the models without changes to minimize horizontal transmission as well [37]. As such, a plan to identify and cull positive animals from the herd as well as quarantine and testing to identify and exclude positive imports may be useful. Methods to control horizontal transmission would likely also be necessary. Clearly, if *Neospora* is already common in the herd, quarantine and testing alone will be ineffective in controlling disease. The results of these models [37] are con-sistent with observational field studies, however further observational and experimental research is needed to confirm their findings before clear recom-mendations can be made.

Environmental control

Mathematical modeling of *Neospora* infection in dairy herds suggests that control of environmental sources of horizontal transmission may be necessary to eradicate disease from a herd [37]. If canine feces are a signifi-cant source of infection for cows then environmental controls to minimize exposure may be prudent. Dogs and wild canids should be prevented from consuming placenta and fetal tissues from abortions. Placentas and fetuses should be collected and disposed of as promptly as possible. Cattle feed sources should be protected from dogs and wild canids to prevent them from defecating in feed.

Vaccination

No vaccine is currently commercially available in the US. Immunogenicity studies on an experimental vaccine has been published [4] but efficacy was not demonstrated following experimental challenge [5]. A Neospora vaccine with a conditional approval exists (Intervet Inc. Millsboro, DE) although no efficacy data from experimental studies or controlled clinical trials are available. A decrease in abortions in a dairy herd following vaccination has been reported, however there was no control group and the criteria for allocation of cows to different vaccination schedules was unclear [24]. A vaccination program would complicate differentiation of naturally infected animals from vaccinates and limit culling options. Clearly more research on the effectiveness of vaccination is required.

Summary

Application of rational principles of risk management in designing an effective biosecurity plan for reproductive diseases can be an important part of a profitable operation. Knowledge of the disease status of the particular herd, the effective strategies for disease exclusion including test performance and reservoirs is necessary. Vaccination can be an effective part of a biosecurity program by increasing herd immunity and decreasing the impact of an outbreak, but by itself will not prevent infections and losses. A more comprehensive approach to disease control is needed. Development and implementation of a biosecurity program is an individualized effort undertaken for a particular operation. Knowledge of the disease status of the herd for each agent of concern and prioritization of the diseases most important in the herd is necessary. The biosecurity plan is then specific for the herd and the particular agent(s) of concern. Practitioners can apply knowledge of the epidemiology and ecology of disease agents to identify and implement logical control points for the individual herd. Many control strategies may be effective for more than one disease. A comprehensive look at the operation is necessary to make sure that the cost of the biosecurity plan does not exceed the return in prevented disease and increased production over the planning period.

References

[1] Allan PJ. A field evaluation of vaccination of bulls against bovine vibriosis. Aust Vet J 1972;48:72–3.
[2] Alt DP, Zuerner RL, Bolin CA. Evaluation of antibiotics for treatment of cattle infected with Leptospira borgpetersenii serovar hardjo. J Am Vet Med Assoc 2001;219:636–9.

[3] Anderson ML, Blanchard PC, Barr BC, et al. *Neospora*-like protozoan infection as a major cause of abortion in California dairy herds. J Am Vet Med Assoc 1991;198:241–4.

[4] Andrianarivo AG, Choromanski L, McDonough SP, et al. Immunogenicity of a killed whole *Neospora caninum* tachyzoite preparation formulated with different adjuvants. Int J Parasitol 1999;29:1613–25.

[5] Andrianarivo AG, Rowe JD, Barr BC, et al. A POLYGEN™-adjuvanted killed *Neospora caninum* tachyzoite preparation failed to prevent foetal infection in pregnant cattle following i.v./i.m. experimental tachyzoite challenge. Int J Parasitol 2000;30:985–90.

[6] Barber JS, Gasser RB, Ellis J, et al. Prevalence of antibodies to *Neospora caninum* in different canid populations. J Parasitol 1997;83:1056–8.

[7] Barling KS, Sherman M, Peterson MJ, et al. Spatial associations among density of cattle, abundance of wild canids, and seroprevalence to *Neospora caninum* in a population of beef calves. J Am Vet Med Assoc 2000;217:1361–5.

[8] Barr BC, BonDurant RH. Viral diseases of the fetus. In: Younquist RS, editor. Current therapy in large animal theriogenology. Philadelphia: WB Saunders; 1997.

[9] Barr BC, Anderson ML. Infectious diseases causing bovine abortion and fetal loss. Vet Clin North Am Food An Pract 1993;9:343–68.

[10] Berg RL, Firehammer BD. Effect of interval between booster vaccination and time of breeding on protection against campylobacteriosis (vibriosis) in cattle. J Am Vet Med Assoc 1978;173:467–71.

[11] Bielanski A, Surujballi O, Thomas EG, et al: Sanitary status of oocytes and embryos collected from heifers experimentally exposed to *Leptospira borgpetersenii* serovar *hardjo-bovis.* Anim Reprod Sci 1998;54:65–73.

[12] Bielanski A, Surujballi O. Association of Leptospira borgpetersenii serovar hardjo type hardjobovis with bovine ova and embryos produced by in-vitro fertilization. Theriogenology 1996;46:45–55.

[13] Bjorkman C, Johansson O, Stenlund S, et al. *Neospora* species infection in a herd of dairy cattle. J Am Vet Med Assoc 1996;208:1441–3.

[14] Bolin CA. Alt DP: Use of a monovalent leptospiral vaccine to prevent renal colonization and urinary shedding in cattle exposed to *Leptospira borgpetersinii* serovar hardjo. Am J Vet Res 2001;62:995–1000.

[15] Bolin CA, Prescott JF. Leptospirosis. In: Howard JL, Smith RA, editors. Current veterinary therapy 4: food animal practice. Philadelphia: WB Saunders; 1999. p. 352–8.

[16] Bolin CA, Thiermann AB, Handsaker AL, et al. Effect of vaccination with a pentavalent leptospiral vaccine on *Leptospira interrogans* serovar *hardjo* type hardjo-bovis infection of pregnant cattle. Am J Vet Res 1989;50:161–5.

[17] Bolin CA, Zuerner RL, Trueba G. Comparison of three techniques to detect *Leptospira interrogans* serovar *hardjo* type hardjo-bovis in bovine urine. Am J Vet Res 1989;50:1001–3.

[18] Bolin CA, Zuerner RL, Trueba G. Effect of vaccination with a pentavalent leptospiral vaccine containing *Leptospira interrogans* serovar *hardjo* type hardjo-bovis on type hardjo-bovis infection of cattle. Am J Vet Res 1989;50:2004–8.

[19] BonDurant RH, Anderson ML, Blanchard P, et al. Prevalence of trichomoniasis among California beef herds. J Am Vet Med Assoc 1990;196:1590–3.

[20] BonDurant RH, Gajadhar A, Campero CM, et al. Preliminary characterization of a *Tritrichomonas foetus*-like protozoan isolated from preputial smega of virgin bulls. Bov Pract 1999;332:124–7.

[21] Bouters R, DeKeyser J, Vandeplassche M, et al. Vibrio fetus infection in bulls: curative and preventive vaccination. Br Vet J 1973;129:52–6.

[22] Buxton D, Maley SW, Pastoret PP, et al. Examination of red foxes (*Vulpes vulpes*) from Belgium for antibody to *Neospora caninum* and *Toxoplasma gondii.* Vet Rec 1997;141:308–9.

[23] Carlsson U, Belak K. Border disease virus transmitted to sheep and cattle by a persistently infected ewe: epidemiology and control. Acta Vet Scand 1994;35:79–98.

[24] Choromanski L, Zimmerman J, Rodgers S. Evaluation of the field performance of the first commercial *Neospora* vaccine in dairy cattle. In: Proceedings 34th Annual Convention of the American Association of Bovine Practitioners, Vancouver, 2001. p. 149.

[25] Clark BL, Dufty JH, Monsbourgh MJ, et al. A duel vaccine for immunisation of bulls against bovine vibriosis. Aust Vet J 1979;55:43.

[26] Clark BL, Dufty JH, Monsbourgh MJ, et al. Immunisation against bovine vibriosis. Vaccination of bulls against infection with Campylobacter fetus subsp venerealis. Aust Vet J 1974;50:407–9.

[27] Clark BL, Fitzpatrick DH. Immunisation against bovine vibriosis. 3. Vaccination against bovine vibriosis in a commercial beef herd in Victoria. Aust Vet J 1972;48:385–7.

[28] Cortese VS, Grooms DL, Ellis J, et al. Protection of pregnant cattle and their fetuses against infection with bovine viral diarrhea virus type 1 by use of a modified-live virus vaccine. Am J Vet Res 1998;59:1409–13.

[29] Cravens RL, Ellsworth MA, Sorensen CD, et al. Efficacy of a temperature-sensitive modified-live bovine herpesvirus type-1 vaccine against abortion and stillbirth in pregnant heifers. J Am Vet Med Assoc 1996;208:2031–4.

[30] Davison HC, French NP, Trees AJ. Herd-specific and age-specific seroprevalence of *Neospora caninum* in 14 British dairy herds. Vet Rec 1999;144:547–50.

[31] Davison HC, Otter O, Trees AJ. Estimation of vertical and horizontal transmission parameters of *Neospora caninum* infections in dairy cattle. Int J Parasitol 1999b;29: 1683–9.

[32] Dekeyser PJ. Bovine genital Campylobacteriosis. In: Morrow DA, Smith RA, editors. Current therapy in theriogenology. Philadelphia: WB Saunders; 1986. p. 263–6.

[33] Dhaliwal GS, Murray RD, Dobson H, et al. Effect of vaccination against *Leptospira interrogans* serovar *hardjo* on milk production and fertility in dairy cattle. Vet Rec 1996;138: 334–5.

[34] Dijsktra Th, Eysker M, Schares G, et al. Dogs shed *Neospora caninum* oocysts after ingestion of naturally infected bovine placenta but not after ingestion of colostrum spiked with *Neospora caninum* tachyzoites. Int J Parasit 2001;31:747–52.

[35] Dubey JP, Hollis K, Romand S, et al. High prevalence of antibodies to *Neospora caninum* in white tailed deer (*Odocoileus virginianus*). Int J Parasitol 1999;29:1709–11.

[36] Fivaz BH, Swanepoel R, McKenzie RL, et al. Passive transmission *of Campylobacter fetus* by immunised bulls. Aus Vet J 1978;54:531–3.

[37] French NP, Clancy D, Davison HC, et al. Mathematical models of *Neospora caninum* infection in dairy cattle: transmission and options for control. Int J Parasitol 1999;29: 1691–704.

[38] Gay JM, Ebel ED, Kearley WP. Commingled grazing as a risk factor for trichomonosis in beef herds. J Am Vet Med Assoc 1996;209:643–6.

[39] Grotelueschen DM, Cheney J, Hudson DB, et al. Bovine trichomoniasis: results of a slaughter survey in Colorado and Nebraska. Theriogenology 1994;42:165–71.

[40] Guitian J, Thurmond MC, Hietala SK. Infertility and abortion among first-lactation dairy cows seropositive or seronegative for *Leptospira interrogans* serovar *hardjo*. J Am Vet Med Assoc 1999;215:515–8.

[41] Gummow B, Myburgh JG, Thompson PN, et al. Three case studies involving *Leptospira interrogans* serovar *pomona* infection in mixed farming units. J S Afr Vet Assoc 1999;70: 29–34.

[42] Hassig M, Lubsen J. relationship between abortions and seroprevalence to selected infectious agents in dairy cows. Journal of Veterinary Medicine Series B 1998;45:435–41.

[43] Heinemann MB, Garcia JF, Nunes CM, et al. Detection and differentiation of *Leptospira* ssp. serovars in bovine semen by polymerase chain reaction and restriction fragment length polymorphism. Vet Microbiol 2000;73:261–7.

[44] Hoar BR, Ribble CS, Spitzer CC, et al. Investigation of pregnancy losses in beef cattle herds associated with *Neospora* sp. Infection. Can Vet J 1996;37:364–6.

[45] Hoerlein AB, Carroll EJ, Kramer T, et al. Bovine vibriosis immunization. J Am Vet Med Assoc 1965;146:828–35.

[46] Houe H. Epidemiology of bovine viral diarrhea virus. Vet Clin North Am Food Anim Pract 1995;11:521–47.

[47] Houe H, Baker JC, Maes RK, et al. Application of antibody titers against bovine viral diarrhea virus (BVDV) as a measure to detect herds with cattle persistently infected with BVDV. J Vet Diagn Invest 1995;7:327–32.

[48] Hum S, Quinn C, Kennedy D. Failure of therapeutic vaccination of a bull infected with Campylobacter fetus. Aust Vet J 1993;70:386–7.

[49] Hum S, Brunner J, McInnes A, et al. Evaluation of cultural methods and selective media for the isolation of *Campylobacter fetus* subsp *venerealis* from cattle. Aust Vet J 1994;71: 184–6.

[50] Kirkbride CA. Leptospiral abortion. In: Kirkbride CA, editor. In: Laboratory diagnosis of livestock abortion, 3rd edition. Ames (IA): Iowa State University Press.

[51] Kirkbride CA. Viral agents and associated lesions detected in a 10-year study of bovine abortions and stillbirths. J Vet Diag Invest 1992;4:374–9.

[52] Kirkbride CA. Bacterial agents detected in a 10-year study of bovine abortions and stillbirths. J Vet Diag Invest 1993;5:64–8.

[53] Kirkland PD, Richards SG, Rothwell JT, et al. Replication of bovine viral diarrhoea virus in the bovine reproductive tract and excretion of virus in semen during acute and chronic infections. Vet Rec 1991;128:587–90.

[54] Kvasnicka WG, Taylor REL, Huang JC, et al. Investigations of the incidence of bovine trichomoniasis in Nevada and of the efficacy of immunizing cattle with vaccines containing *Tritrichomonas foetus*. Theriogenology 1989;31:963–71.

[55] Kvasnicka WG, Hanks D, Huang J, et al. Clinical evaluation of the efficacy of inoculating cattle with a vaccine containing *Tritrichomonas foetus*. Am J Vet Res 1992;53:2023–7.

[56] Kvasnicka WG, Hall M, Hanks D. Current concepts in the control of Bovine Trichomoniasis. Compend Cont Educ Pract Vet 1996;18:S105–11.

[57] Lang-Ree JR, Vatn T, Kommisrud E, et al. Transmission of bovine viral diarrhoea by rectal examination. Vet Rec 1994;135:412–3.

[58] Lindsay DS, Dubey JP, Duncan RB. Confirmation that the dog is a definitive host for *Neospora caninum.*. Vet Parasit 1999;82:327–33.

[59] Lindsay DS, Kelly EJ, McKown RD, et al. Prevalence of *Neospora caninum* and *Toxoplasma gondii* antibodies in coyotes (*Canis latrans*) and experimental infections of coyotes with *Neospora caninum.*. J Parasitol 1996;82:657–9.

[60] Little TWA, Hathaway SC, Broughton ES, et al. Control of *Leptospira hardjo* infection in beef cattle by whole herd vaccination. Vet Rec 1992;131:90–2.

[61] Loken T. Ruminant pestivirus infections in animals other than cattle and sheep. Vet Clin North Am Food An Pract 1995;11:597–614.

[62] Mars MH, Bruschke CJM, Oirschot JT, et al. Airborne transmission of BHV1 (bovine herpesvirus 1). BRSV (bovine respiratory virus), and BVDV (bovine viral diarrhoea virus) among cattle is possible under experimental conditions. Vet Micro 1999;66:197–207.

[63] McAllister MM, Huffman EM, Hietala SK, et al. Evidence suggesting a point source exposure in an outbreak of bovine abortion due to neosporosis. J Vet Diagn Invest 1996;8:355–7.

[64] McAllister MM, Dubey JP, Lindsay DS, et al. Dogs are definitive hosts for *Neospora caninum.*. Int J Parasitol 1998;28:1473–8.

[65] McAllister MM, Bjorkman C, Anderson-Sprecher R, et al. Evidence of a point source exposure to *Neospora caninum* and protective immunity in a herd of beef cows. J Am Vet Med Assoc 2000;217:881–7.

[66] McGowan MR, Kirkland PD, Rodwell BJ, et al. A field investigation of the effects of bovine viral diarrhea virus infection around the time of insemination on the reproductive performance of cattle. Theriogenology 1993;39:443–9.

[67] McGuire AM, McAllister M, Wills RA, et al. Experimental inoculation of domestic pigeons (*Columbia livia*) and zebra finches (*Poephila guttata*) with *Neospora caninum* tachyzoites. Int J Parasitol 1999;29:1525–9.

[68] Merien F, Amouriaux P, Perolat P, et al. Polymerase chain reaction for detection of *Leptospira* ssp. in clinical samples. J Clin Micrbiol 1992;30:2219–24.

[69] Meyling A, Ronsholt L, Dalsgaard K. et al. Experimental exposure of vaccinated and non-vaccinated pregnant cattle to isolates of bovine viral diarrhoea virus (BVDV). In: Agriculture–pestivirus infections of ruminants. Luxembourg: Office for Official Publications of the European Communities; 1987. p. 225–31.

[70] Miller DA, Wilson MA, Beran GW. Survey to estimate prevalence of *Leptospira interrogans* infection in mature cattle in the United States. Am J Vet Res 1991;52:1761–5.

[71] Miller DA, Wilson MA, Beran GW. Relationship between prevalence of *Leptospira interrogans* in cattle, and regional climatic, and seasonal factors. Am J Vet Res 1991;52:1766–8.

[72] Monke DR, Mitchell JR. Risk analysis: CSS testing protocol for Trichomoniasis. In: Proceedings of the 17th Technical Conference on Artificial Insemination & Reproduction. Middleton (WI); 1998. p. 37–42.

[73] Nettleton PF. Pestivirus infections in ruminants other that cattle. Res Sci tech Off Int Epiz 1990;9:131–50.

[74] Njaa BL, Edward GC, Janzen E, et al. Diagnosis of persistent bovine viral diarrhea virus infection by immunohistochemical staining or formalin-fixed skin biopsy specimens. J Vet Diagn Invest 2000;12:393–9.

[75] Osorio FA. Infectious bovine rhinotracheitis and other clinical syndromes caused by bovine herpes virus types 1 and 5. In: Howard JL, Smith RA, editors. In: Current veterinary therapy 4 food animal practice. Philadelphia: WB Saunders; 1999.

[76] Pare JP. Thurmond MC Hietala SK: Congenital *Neospora caninum* infection in dairy cattle and associated calfhood mortality. Can J Vet Res 1996;60:133–9.

[77] Pare JP, Fecteau G, Fortin M, et al. Seroepidemiologic study of *Neospora caninum* in dairy herds. J Am Vet Med Assoc 1998;213:1595–8.

[78] Quintanilla-Gozalo A, Pereira-Bueno J, Tabares E, et al. Seroprevalence of *Neospora caninum* infection in dairy and beef cattle in Spain. Internatl. J. Parasitol. 1999;29:1201–8.

[79] Rae DO. Impact of trichomoniasis on the cow-calf producer's profitability. J Am Vet Med Assoc 1989;194:771–5.

[80] Rae DO, Chenoweth PJ, Genho PC, et al. Prevalence of Tritrichomonas fetus in a bull population and effect on production in a large cow-calf enterprise. J Am Vet Med Assoc 1999;214:1051–5.

[81] Sanderson MW, Gay JM. Veterinary involvement in management practices of beef cow-calf producers. J Am Vet Med Assoc 1996;208:488–91.

[82] Sanderson MW, Dargatz DA, Garry FB. Biosecurity practices of beef cow-calf producers. J Am Vet Med Assoc 2000;217:185–9.

[83] Sanderson MW, Gay JM, Baszler TV. *Neospora caninum* seroprevalence and associated risk factors in beef cattle in the northwestern United States. Vet. Parasit 2000;90:15–24.

[84] Sandvik T, Krogsrud J. Evaluation of an antigen-capture ELISA for detection of bovine viral diarrhea virus in cattle blood samples. J Vet Diagn Invest 1995;7:65–71.

[85] Sandvik T. Laboratory diagnostic investigations for bovine viral diarrhoea virus infections in cattle. Vet Microbiol 1999;64:123–34.

[86] Schurig GG, Duncan JR, Winter AJ. Elimination of genital vibriosis in femal cattle by systemic immunization with killed cells or cell-free extracts of Campylobacter fetus. J Infect Dis 1978;138:463–72.

[87] Skirrow SZ. Identification of trichomonad carrier cows. J Am Vet Med Assoc 1987;191:553–4.

[88] Smith DR. Epidemiologic tools for biosecurity and biocontainment. Vet Clin North Am Food An Pract 2002;18:155–73.

[89] Stewart RJE, Campbell JR, Janzen ED, et al. The effects of *Tritrichomonas foetus* and nutritional status on the fertility of cows on a community pasture. Can Vet J 1998;39: 638–41.

[90] Tarry DW, Bernal L, Edwards S. Transmission of bovine virus diarrhoea by blood feeding flies. Vet Rec 1991;128:182–4.

[91] Tessaro SV, Carman PS, Deregt D. Viremia and virus shedding in elk infected with type 1 and virulent type 2 bovine viral diarrhea virus. J Wild Dis 1999;35:671–7.

[92] Thur B, Zlinszky K, Ehrensperger F. Immunohistochemical detection of bovine viral diarrhea virus in skin biopsies: a reliable and fast diagnostic tool. J Vet Med B 1996;43: 163–6.

[93] Thurmond MC, Picanso JP, Hietala SK. Prospective serology and analysis in diagnosis of dairy cow abortion. J Vet Diag Invest 1990;2:274–82.

[94] Thurmond MC, Hietala SK. Culling associated with Neospora caninum infection in dairy cows. Am J Vet Res 1996;57:1559–62.

[95] Thurmond MC, Hietala SK. Effect of *Neospora caninum* infection on milk production in first lactation dairy cows. J Am Vet Med Assoc 1997a;210:672–4.

[96] Thurmond MC, Hietala SK, Blanchard PC. Herd-based diagnosis of *Neospora caninum*-induced endemic and epidemic abortion in cows and evidence for congenital and postnatal transmission. J Vet Diag Invest 1997;9:44–9.

[97] Uggla A, Stenlund S, Holmdahl OJM, et al. Oral *Neospora caninum* inoculation of neonatal calves. Int J Parasitol 1998;28:1467–72.

[98] Vasquez LA, Ball L, Bennett BW, et al. Bovine genital campylobacteriosis (vibriosis): vaccination of experimentally infected bulls. Am J Vet Res 1983;44:1553–7.

[99] Waldner CL, Janzen ED, Ribble CS. Determination of the association between *Neospora caninum* infection and reproductive performance in beef herds. J Am Vet Med Assoc 1998;213:685–90.

[100] Waldner CL, Janzen ED, Henderson J, et al. Outbreak of abortion associated with *Neospora caninum* infection in a beef herd. J Am Vet Med Assoc 1999;215:1485–90.

[101] Walker RL. Bovine venereal Campylobacteriosis. In: Howard JL, Smith RA, editors. In: Current veterinary therapy 4 food animal practice. St Louis: Mosby.

[102] Wikse SE, Baker JC. The Bronchopneumonias. In: Smith BP, Smith RA, editors. Large animal internal medicine. Philadelphia: WB Saunders; 1999. p. 352–8.

[103] Williams DJL, Guy CS, McGarry JW, et al. *Neospora caninum*-associated abortion in cattle: the time of experimentally-induced parasitaemia during gestation determined foetal survival. Parasitology 2000;121:347–58.

[104] Wouda W, Moen AR, Schukken YH. Abortion risk in progeny of cows after a *Neospora caninum* epidemic. Theriogenology 1998;49:1311–6.

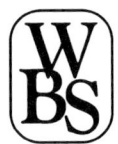

THE VETERINARY
CLINICS
Food Animal
Practice

Vet Clin Food Anim 18 (2002) 99–114

Biosecurity for arthropod-borne diseases

Brian J. McCluskey, DVM, MS

*United States Department of Agriculture, Animal and Plant Health Inspection Service,
Veterinary Services, Centers for Epidemiology and Animal Health,
555 South Howes Street, Fort Collins, CO 80521, USA*

A wide range of diseases or disorders of cattle are caused directly by arthropods. Infestations with *Hypoderma* spp. (grubs), lice, ticks, or mites can result in damage to hides, blood loss, and poor weight gain. Harassment by swarms of biting flies results in fatigue and reductions in feed intake with subsequent loss of production.

The focus of this article is on pathogens transmitted either mechanically or biologically to cattle by arthropods, not on the effects of the arthropods themselves. Mechanical transmission of disease involves the physical movement of a pathogen from one animal to another without extensive replication of the pathogen in the vector or effect of the pathogen on the arthropod vector. The face fly (*Musca autumnalis*) prefers the area around the eyes, mouth, and muzzle of cattle and may acquire *Moraxella bovis* bacteria, one factor in infectious bovine keratoconjunctivitis, from infected cattle and move the bacteria to other cattle. Although the fly may carry the bacteria for up to 3 days, there is little replication of the bacteria in the fly itself [14]. Biologic transmission requires multiplication of a pathogen in the arthropod or that a stage of the pathogen's life cycle occurs in one or more arthropod species. Bluetongue virus, present in insect-ingested blood, replicates in the midgut cells of *Culicoides* spp. The transmission cycle in the *Culicoides* spp. requires 10 to 15 days. Although the appropriate use of insecticides may play a critical role in the control of arthropod-borne diseases (ABDs), an understanding of vector, pathogen, and host biology and ecology is integral to the prevention and control of ABDs on cattle operations.

The best example of control of an ABD is the eradication of Texas cattle fever or babesiosis from the United States. *Babesia bigemina*, the causative

---

E-mail address: Brian.J.Mccluskey@aphis.usda.gov

agent of this disease, is transmitted by an intermediate arthropod host, *Boophilus annulatus*. The classical investigations of Smith and Kilbourne established the life cycle of the protozoan parasite. Tick vector eradication was the cornerstone of Texas cattle fever control and was accomplished by dipping cattle every 2 to 3 weeks in dip tanks filled with arsenical acaricides [10]. Today a wide variety of improved acaricides are available, including chlorinated hydrocarbons, carbamates, and organophosphates, and disease remains limited to occasional incursions across the Mexico–US border into Texas.

Ecology

Vector ecology

The risk of transmission of an arthropod-borne pathogen to cattle is primarily associated with the density and competency of insect vectors. Vector density is influenced by climatic factors, including temperature, precipitation, and humidity. For example, cases of vesicular stomatitis, an arthropod-borne viral disease of livestock, were shown to be associated with the total monthly precipitation that occurred 10 to 12 months prior to reported cases (Brian J. McCluskey, DVM, MS, unpublished data, 2001). It was hypothesized that above-average precipitation during the vector season might provide larger numbers of potential breeding sites, and therefore, larger populations of arthropod vectors in the next transmission season. Populations of *Culicoides* spp., which are associated with the transmission of bluetongue viruses, are also intimately linked to meteorologic conditions. Inadequate rainfall inhibits *Culicoides* larval development, and copious rainfall may cause a washing out of the best larval development sites, resulting in population suppression [5]. Understanding the differences in arthropod breeding cycles and habitats is imperative in developing control strategies. For example, black flies (*Simulidae*) require slow- to fast-moving streams for development, whereas most *Culicoides* species prefer muddy areas or those with high levels of organic matter for oviposition and development. Temperature also has been shown to affect fecundity and development of *Culicoides* spp [9].

Vector competence is also a primary factor in the risk of disease transmission. An effective arthropod vector must support the pathogen it is transmitting. Vector competence for mechanical transmission is limited to the insect's ability to acquire the pathogen by blood meal or simple contact and move the pathogen to another host quickly enough that the pathogen survives transport. The pathogen does not multiply in this situation, but a physical or chemical bond does occur to allow for survival during transport. Competence is primarily associated with biologic vectors in which the vector provides a specific medium for the replication or development of the pathogen. The insect gut often is an important barrier that must be crossed for complete development to occur, with an infectious pathogen eventually moving to the salivary gland. These specific insect characteristics determine which arthropods transmit disease and which do not. Insect density, vector competence, and the availability of a susceptible host are the primary but not sole determinants of pathogen transmission.

Longevity of vectors is required for transmission as well. Many arthropods have developed overwintering mechanisms or vertical transmission that sustains pathogens in insect populations. More short-term longevity is required when multiple feedings of arthropods are needed for transmission. The period from pathogen acquisition to transfer to a susceptible host requires a specific amount of time for development of the pathogen to an infective stage in the gut or salivary glands. Feeding frequency and timing, vector mobility or flight ranges, and vector adaptability to environmental conditions, including the application of insecticides, are additional determinants of pathogen transmission [6].

Pathogen ecology

Pathogens develop various survival mechanisms to move from one infected host to another. These mechanisms are as complex as the trans-stadial transmission of *Anaplasma marginale* in *Dermacentor* spp. of ticks to the short-term (<1 h) survival of bovine leukosis virus on the mouthparts of stable flies (*Stomoxys calcitrans*) and horn flies (*Haematobia irritans*) [1]. A requirement for any infectious agent to survive is a mechanism for transmission from one host to another. Disease-transmission modeling assumes that infection is spread from infected individuals to susceptible individuals by adequate contact between the two hosts [12]. Vectorial capacity is a mathematical estimation of the probability of effective contact and defines the number of potentially infective bites that will ultimately occur by all vectors feeding on a single susceptible host in 1 day [4]. An arthropod-borne pathogen's transmission success is therefore dependent on the vectorial capacity. It is the complex relationship of pathogen, vector, and host that determines effective contact and where and when disease will occur.

Host ecology

Hosts do not remain passive to attacks of insect vectors or to the pathogens carried by those vectors. Physical avoidance, including tail switching, ear flapping, and skin twitching, are simple but marginally effective methods used to defend against insect attack. Immersing in water, coating with mud, or crowding together are other physical avoidance techniques used specifically by cattle. Numerous immunologic defense mechanisms also are used against ABDs. It is beyond the scope of this article to discuss the multiple components of the bovine immune system that defend against pathogen incursions; however, all of these components play an integral role in the defense against arthropod-borne pathogens.

Arthropod-borne diseases of North America

Table 1 provides a list of some common ABDs of cattle in North America. Vectors include hematophagous flies, nonhematophagous flies, and tick species. Pathogen types include protozoans, bacteria, viruses, and rickettsial agents. The geographic distribution of these diseases is dependent on the vector, pathogen, and host ecologic factors discussed previously. For example, occurrence of enzootic bovine abortion has been limited to areas of northern California, Nevada, and Oregon, although the distribution of the disease seems to be expanding [11]. Although the causative agent of this disease has not been identified, it appears that the disease's limited distribution is owing to the specific ecologies of the vector (*Ornithodoros coriaceus*) and the pathogen. Contrasting enzootic bovine abortion with bovine leukosis infections, one finds a much wider geographic distribution of disease. The National Animal Health Monitoring System Dairy 1996 study [1] found that 89% of US dairy operations had cattle that were seropositive for bovine leukosis virus. Prevalences in the West, Midwest, and Northeast were 87% to 89%, whereas in the southeast region a herd prevalence of 99% was estimated. These high prevalences are not solely attributable to arthropod transmission, but the arthropods suggested to be associated with transmission of bovine leukosis virus (stable flies, horn flies, and tabanids) are found throughout the United States.

Table 1
Important arthropod-borne diseases of cattle in North America

Disease	Pathogen	Vector type	Vector species
Anaplasmosis	*Anaplasma marginale*	Ticks (primarily)	*Boophilus* spp *Dermacentor* spp *Ixodes* spp *Rhipicephalus* spp
Anthrax	*Bacillus anthracis*	Hematophagous flies	Many
Babesiosis	*Babesia bigemina*	Tick	*Boophilus* spp
Bluetongue	Bluetongue virus	Hematophagous flies	*Culicoides* spp
Bovine leukosis	Bovine leukemia virus	Hematophagous flies	Tabanids *Stomoxys calcitrans*
Enzootic bovine abortion *coriaceous*	Unknown	Tick	*Ornithodoros*
Lyme disease	*Borrelia burgdorferi*	Tick	*Ixodes* spp
Infectious bovine keratoconjunctivitis	*Moraxella bovis*	Nonbiting flies	*Musca* spp *Stomoxys calcitrans*
Vesicular stomatitis	Vesicular stomatitis virus	Hematophagous flies	*Lutzyomia* spp *Simulium* spp *Culicoides* spp
		Nonbiting flies	Many

Biosecurity risk assessment

The development of biosecurity plans on cattle operations should focus on specific strategies that prevent introduction of pathogens to the operation and control spread of pathogens already present on the operation. Risk-assessment techniques are proposed as appropriate tools for the development of biosecurity practices on cattle operations, and the risk-assessment framework is used herein to outline the approaches to biosecurity for ABDs [16]. The descriptions of vector, pathogen, and host ecology and discussion of typical ABDs in North America provided in previous sections of this article were necessary because they are the inputs for the risk assessment.

Hazard identification

The development of biosecurity protocols specific to ABDs requires the initial identification of the diseases that are most likely to affect the operation in question. As mentioned previously, for some ABDs, their widespread geographic distribution requires that they be included in all operations' lists of potential hazards. For example, infectious bovine keratoconjunctivitis and bovine leukosis virus and the vectors that transmit them are ubiquitous and should be considered potential hazards on all cattle operations. In contrast, the potential for the occurrence of babesiosis is limited strictly to those operations at risk of exposure to the tick vectors of the pathogen (e.g., the southern tier of Texas). The occurrence of clinical cases of vesicular stomatitis has been limited to southwestern states since the 1980s, so it is unlikely, for example, that a dairy in northern New York would be at risk for natural exposure to the known vesicular stomatitis viruses.

In addition to identification of the pathogens, the potential economic losses to the operation from each pathogen must be considered. Bovine leukosis has been shown to affect production on dairy operations and is a disease that may affect marketing of animals and germplasm, but the costs of prevention and control should be compared with those potential losses before instituting controls [8]. It may be of little financial benefit to a commercial dairyman to initiate testing and culling, extensive insect abatement, and other controls for bovine leukosis virus, whereas the identical program may be imperative for a dairyman with registered cattle who exports embryos internationally.

Exposure assessment

After identification of potential hazards, the next step in the development of biosecurity plans for ABDs requires assessment of how cattle might be exposed to the identified pathogens. ABDs can enter an operation or move among groups on an operation by introduction of an infected animal, presenting the carrier vector with the agent or both concurrently. Once the pathogen and arthropod are established on the operation, then the disease cycle is initiated. As is typical for many pathogens, including those transmitted by arthropods, the addition of new animals to an operation is the initial method of introduction. For example, cattle infected with *Anaplasma marginale* remain carriers for years, and outbreaks generally occur when carrier animals are introduced into naive herds [3]. The introduction of bovine leukosis virus can occur similarly.

An exposure assessment for the introduction of vesicular stomatitis virus (VSV) would not find new additions to a herd as a key risk factor. Latent infections, a viremic state, and carrier animals have not been identified in the epidemiology of vesicular stomatitis. Only cattle with active lesions are capable of transmitting the virus. It is therefore highly unlikely that a healthy new addition will introduce VSV to an operation, and other modes of introduction should be considered. Epidemiologic and experimental studies provide evidence that VSV is transmitted by arthropods in the southwestern United States [7,13]. A case-control study found that the risk of a premises housing animals that tested positive for vesicular stomatitis was 2.6 times greater on premises that housed their livestock within 0.25 miles of a source of running water [7]. Black flies (*Simulidae*) are a primary vector candidate of VSV in the southwestern United States, and as mentioned previously, require slow-moving streams or irrigation ditches for their oviposition and development. This information, in combination with knowledge of the flight ranges of the black flies, is a key exposure factor to investigate on operations in areas where vesicular stomatitis occurs. Similarly, for enzootic bovine abortion, if an operation has cattle that graze in northern California, southern Oregon, or western Nevada, the grazing area should be examined for typical tick habitats.

Risk characterization

After identification of the potential hazards (pathogen and disease) and assessment of the modes of exposure of cattle to the potential hazards, the level of exposure risk must be estimated. Qualitative estimation of risk is generally adequate in the development of biosecurity protocols. Information regarding when and where an operation acquires replacements is probably more important than knowing precisely how many replacements were purchased from each source. Information about the natural history of anthrax in the area around the cattle operation is more important than a geospatial analysis of anthrax outbreaks. Practitioners and producers often conduct qualitative estimations of exposure risks informally and then mutually decide on acceptable approaches to prevention or control. A more formal characterization of risks may simply require development of a checklist to use while conducting a walk-through of the operation. The exposure assessment and risk characterizations can be included on the same checklist.

Mitigations

The aim of these types of qualitative risk assessments is to identify mitigations that lessen the risk of disease introduction or spread on a cattle operation. Prevention and control of arthropods, whether to prevent their inherent adverse effects or to eliminate the pathogens they may transmit, have historically been accomplished through the application of insecticides. This singular approach often has proven unsatisfactory, and in many cases has resulted in exacerbating the development of insecticide resistance. Integrated pest management programs consider biologic and habitat controls as well as insecticide use, maximizing the effectiveness of insecticides applied [15].

Habitat control is dependent on a thorough understanding of the biology and ecology of potential disease vectors. For example, the two primary vectors of *Moraxella bovis*, the house fly and the stable fly, breed in manure piles, decaying vegetation, and other organic matter. Waste management is a key mitigation in reducing fly populations. Elimination of potential breeding sites is accomplished through removal of manure, bedding, and uneaten feed and ensuring proper drainage of stalls. For a disease such as vesicular stomatitis, habitat control is more tenuous. The host's habitat, not the vector's, must be altered. The elimination of sources of running water, which serve as the breeding and development sites for black flies, may not be feasible if they are used for irrigation or as a source of drinking water. In this case, during a vesicular stomatitis outbreak, removal of cattle from an area near a source of running water during the early evening hours may be the most effective habitat control available. *Culicoides* spp. are also potential vectors of VSVs. Elimination of wet, muddy areas around watering troughs and other areas of standing water may reduce the breeding habitats of *Culicoides* spp.

Biologic controls take advantage of naturally occurring predators of arthropods to reduce the populations of disease vectors. Parasitic wasps are an important biologic control agent for many species of flies. These wasps feed on fly larva, primarily larva found in manure or other organic material, and also lay eggs in the pupa of the flies. In both cases, the fly is killed. It is important to protect these advantageous insects through prudent applications of insecticides. Release of parasitic species also can help in the control of fly populations. It is imperative that the correct species of parasite be selected for the operation's climate and ecology. Research has indicated that the costs associated with fly parasite releases have been offset by reductions in the costs of insecticide applications [15]. Local extension agents can assist in the selection of the appropriate species of fly parasites for each cattle operation.

Chemical controls also must be considered in the integrated approach to insect management. Residual premises sprays, space sprays, larvicides, and insecticides applied to animals are options for chemical control. Tables 2 and 3 list some insecticides available for control of flies on cattle operations. Correct selection, timing of application, and dosing of insecticides avoid the exacerbation of insecticide resistance and the potential for pesticide residues in meat or milk. All label directions should be followed strictly.

Improving host immunity also should be considered in developing biosecurity plans for ABDs. For most of the ABDs listed in Table 1, however, vaccines are either not available or are of questionable efficacy. Commer-

Table 2
Control of flies in and around livestock barns[a]

Method of application	Active ingredient	Examples of trade names[b]
Space spray	Synergized pyrethrins	Several formulations
	Synergized pyrethrins plus permethrin	Several formulations
	Synergized permethrin	Several formulations
	Synergized pyrethrins plus dichlorvos	Py-Vona Stock Fly Spray (several formulations)
Residual premise	Permethrin	Atroban, Ectiban EC (several formulations)
	Synergized pyrethrins plus dichlorvos	Py-Vona Stock Fly Spray
	Synergized resmethrin (remove animals from building)	Syn-Tech 2.5 plus 10% insecticide
	Diazinon (beef barns only; remove animals from building)	Several formulations
	Cyfluthrin (remove animals from building)	Countdown EC (several formulations)
	Chlorpyrifos (remove animals from building)	MEC Chlorpyrifos Livestock Premise Spray Concentrate
	Naled	Dibrom 8
	Dimethoate (remove animals from building)	Cygon (several formulations)
Animal treatment	Permethrin	Atroban, Ectiban EC (several formulations)
Bait	Methomyl	Blue Streak, Golden Malrin, Musca-Cide Fly Bait
Larvicide	Diflubenzuron	Vigilante (bolus)
Larvicide (manure treatment)	Tetrachlorvinphos	Rabon (several formulations)
Larvicide (feed additive)	Tetrachlorvinphos	Rabon (several formulations)
	Methoprene	Altosid Cattle Custom Blending Premix

[a] Read and follow product labels carefully for target pest information, compatibility of treatment with other animal management practices, and precautions to avoid contamination of feed and water.

[b] Trade names are cited for convenience only. Other products with similar active ingredients may be available.

Adapted *from* Rutz DA, Geden CJ, Pitts Cw. Pest management recommendations for dairy cattle. Cornell and Penn State Cooperative Extension Publication, Pennsylvania State University; 2000; with permission [15].

cial anaplasmosis vaccines are currently unavailable, because those used previously were not efficacious and were capable of inducing neonatal isoerythrolysis. Locally produced anaplasmosis vaccines may be available in some states. Administration of anthrax vaccine is restricted to endemic

Table 3
Control of flies on pastured cattle[a]

Method of application	Active ingredient	Examples of trade names[b]
For Use on Lactating Dairy Cattle (also Beef and Nonlactating Dairy Cattle)		
Ear tag	Permethrin	Several formulations
	Fenvalerate	Super Deckem (several formulations)
	Synergized cypermethrin	Python
	Synergized chlorpyrifos plus cypermethrin	Max-Con
	Cyfluthrin	Cutter Gold (several formulations)
Dust	Permethrin	Several formulations
	Tetrachlorvinphos	Rabon (several formulations)
Oil solution in backrubber	Permethrin	Several formulations
Animal spray	Permethrin	Atroban, Ectiban EC (several formulations)
	*Synergized pyrethrins plus dichlorvos	Py-Vona Stock Fly
Spray	Coumaphos (horn fly)	Co-Ral 25% WP
	Naled	Dibrom 8
	Tetrachlorvinphos	Raban (several formulations)
Pour-on	Permethrin	Several formulations
	*Cyfluthrin	Several formulations
	Eprinomectin	Eprinex
Bolus (larvicide)	Diflubenzuron	Vigilante
Feed additive (larvicide)	Tetrachlorvinphos	Rabon (several formulations)
	Methoprene	Altosid Cattle Custom Blending Premix
For Use on Beef and Dairy Young Stock		
Ear tag	Synergized cyhalothrin	Saber Extra
	Cyhalothrin plus pirimiphos-methyl	Double Barrel VP
	Diazinon	X-Terminator, Optimizer
	Pirimiphos-methyl	Dominator
	Diazinon plus chlorpyrifos	Warrior
Dust	Malathion	Several formulations
Oil solution in backrubber	Phosmet	Del-Phos (several formulations)

(continued on next page)

Table 3 (continued)

Method of application	Active ingredient	Examples of trade names[b]
Animal spray	Methoxychlor	Several formulations
Pour-on	Fenthion	Lysoff (several formulations)
	Lambda cyhalothrin	Saber (several formulations)
Larvicide pour-on	Avermectin	Dectomax, Ivomec
Injectable (larvicide)	Avermectin	Ivomec, Dectomax

[a] Read and follow product labels carefully for target pest information, compatibility of treatment with other animal management practices, and precautions to avoid contamination of feed and water.

[b] Trade names are cited for convenience only. Other products with similar active ingredients may be available.

Adapted from Rutz DA, Geden CJ, Pitts Cw. Pest management recommendations for dairy cattle. Cornell and Penn State Cooperative Extension Publication, Pennsylvania State University; 2000; with permission [15].

areas or during anthrax outbreaks, and it is not carried out for general prevention purposes. Cattle vaccines for bluetongue, bovine leukosis virus, enzootic bovine abortion, and Lyme disease are not available. Commercial vaccines are available for infectious bovine keratoconjunctivitis, and autogenous vaccines for VSV have been made available during vesicular stomatitis outbreaks in the southwestern United States.

The animal that is the "new addition" is often the source of disease introduction and must be considered a key risk factor in the development of biosecurity protocols. Pre-testing of new additions for potential ABD can provide some indication of what pathogens are being brought onto the farm. It is important to determine initially the prevalence of diseases of interest currently existing on the operation. Serosurveys can provide indications of previous exposure, and in some cases, levels of immunity to the diseases of interest. Ideally, test results should be received and decisions made about receiving the animals before their arrival on the operation. Placing new additions in isolation while awaiting test results is an appropriate management strategy for many diseases, but it may do little to prevent the spread of ABDs.

Biosecurity practices for arthropods and the diseases they may carry historically focused on the use of insecticides. It is important to understand the ecologies of the arthropods, pathogens, and hosts and integrate the basic principles of disease prevention to design effective biosecurity practices for ABDs on cattle operations. The list provided in the Box below used in two scenarios, presents questions to be answered in the development of biosecurity protocols specific to ABDs. This checklist must be considered simultaneously with the development of general operation-level biosecurity protocols. As mentioned previously, operation managers must also consider the costs and benefits of instituting biosecurity plans designed to prevent the introduction or spread of ABDs. Costs to consider are those associated with production, restrictions on trade, food safety, and the potential to affect

---

Biosecurity risk assessment for arthropod-borne diseases

Hazard identification
  What ABDs are most likely to occur on this operation?
  What are the likely vectors of each disease?
  What are the estimated financial effects on production for each disease?
Exposure assessment
  What are the breeding habitats of the vectors?
  What are the flight ranges of the vectors?
  What are the feeding habits of the vectors?
  Are new cattle added to this herd other than by natural additions?
Risk characterization
  Where are new additions acquired?
  Are new additions tested for any of the diseases listed before arrival on this operation?
  Has there been clinical evidence or specific diagnoses made of any of the diseases listed?
  Are cattle on this operation vaccinated for any of the diseases listed?
  Are there outbreaks or occurrences of any of the diseases listed reported in this operation's area?

---

public health. Exclusion or control of an ABD may be feasible but too costly to warrant implementation.

Two scenarios may help in the application of the risk-assessment framework presented. It is important to recognize that the level of concern for any specific ABD is specific to individual producers, so the biosecurity programs designed would also be highly individualized.

Scenario one

This scenario assumes that the producer of a cow–calf operation in southern Idaho is interested in expanding the herd by 10% and will be buying 50 bred cows this fall.

Hazard identification

What ABDs are most likely to occur on this operation?

Pinkeye, bovine leukosis virus, and anaplasmosis are assumed to be the most likely ABDs to occur on this operation based on the location and production type.

What are the likely vectors of each disease listed above?

Face flies, stable flies, and *Dermacentor* spp. of ticks are the likely vectors of pinkeye, bovine leukosis virus, and anaplasmosis, respectively.

What are the estimated financial effects on production for each disease listed above?

The financial effects of pinkeye and bovine leukosis virus are assumed to be minimal by the operation, whereas the effect of anaplasmosis could be substantial. The biosecurity plan will be developed to prevent and control anaplasmosis.

Exposure assessment

What are the breeding and feeding habitats and habits of the vectors listed above?

The Rocky Mountain wood tick is a three-host tick which, as a subadult, feeds primarily on small rodents; as adults, these ticks focus on large mammals, especially deer, humans, canids, and livestock. They are primarily found on animals.

What are the movement or flight ranges of the vectors listed above?

Movement is minimal other than when attached to hosts.

Are new cattle added to this herd other than by natural additions?

Plans are to add cattle to this herd immediately.

Risk characterization

Where are new additions acquired?

New additions are generally purchased at local livestock markets.

Are new additions tested for any of the diseases listed above before arrival on this operation?

No pre-arrival testing is routinely conducted on new additions.

Has there been clinical evidence or specific diagnoses made of any of the diseases listed above?

A few cases of anaplasmosis have been diagnosed at this operation.

Are cattle on this operation vaccinated for any of the diseases listed above?

Anaplasmosis vaccines are not available.

Are there outbreaks or occurrences of any of the diseases listed above reported in this operation's area?

Anaplasmosis is endemic in this operation's area.

Mitigations

Levels of current infection on the operation can be assessed by serosurvey. Long-acting tetracycline products (200 mg/mL at the rate of 20 mg/kg) can be administered to seropositive animals to treat parasetemias. Examination of cattle for tick infestation should be conducted, and if ticks are observed, all cattle should be treated with an acaricide. The practitioner should avoid using common needles to administer medications or vaccines to cattle, and he or she should clean and disinfect instruments that are used in treatment (e.g., dehorners, implant guns).

Before purchase of cattle to expand the herd, the source and geographic location of cattle to be purchased should be identified. Producers should avoid buying cattle from areas known to be endemic for anaplasmosis. Serologic testing by complement fixation for detection of carrier animals should be conducted. The purchase of seropositive cattle should be avoided, but if it is necessary, then seropositive animals should be treated with long-acting tetracycline formulations.

Scenario two

This scenario considers a 200-cow, closed-herd drylot dairy on the western slope of Colorado where the owners are interested in instituting biosecurity standard operating procedures.

Hazard identification

What ABDs are most likely to occur on this operation?

Pinkeye, bovine leukosis virus, anaplasmosis, and vesicular stomatitis must be considered as ABDs that can occur on this dairy.

What are the likely vectors of each disease listed above?

Face flies, stable flies, *Dermacentor* spp. of ticks, and black flies (*Simulidae*) are the likely vectors of pinkeye, bovine leukosis virus, anaplasmosis, and VSV, respectively.

What are the estimated financial effects on production for each disease listed above?

Bovine leukosis virus and VSV are considered to be the two primary ABDs that may adversely affect production on this dairy. Outbreaks of vesicular stomatitis have occurred in this area sporadically and are of great concern to this producer because of restrictions on movement of cattle and the potential for severe decreases in production caused by oral lesions and cases of mastitis.

Exposure assessment

What are the breeding and feeding habitats and habits of the vectors listed above?

Stable flies lay eggs and develop in rotting organic matter such as manure, old hay, or straw and silage. Stable flies are blood-feeding arthropods. Black flies develop in slow-moving water such as streams and irrigation ditches. Peak feeding times for black flies are typically in the evening hours, and they may live up to 30 days as adults.

What are the movement or flight ranges of the vectors listed above?

Stable flies generally do not fly far from their source of food or breeding sites. Black flies have been reported to have flight ranges of up to 8 miles, although much shorter distances are more common. Reports have been made of black flies traveling on winds for long distances.

Are new cattle added to this herd other than by natural additions?

This is a closed herd, so no new cattle are added.

Risk characterization

Where are new additions acquired?

Not applicable.

Are new additions tested for any of the diseases listed above before arrival on this operation?

Not applicable.

Has there been clinical evidence or specific diagnoses made of any of the diseases listed above?

A few cases of lymphosarcoma in older cows have been diagnosed. No cases of vesicular stomatitis have been diagnosed on this farm.

Are cattle on this operation vaccinated for any of the diseases listed above?

Bovine leukosis virus vaccines are not available, and the autogenous VSV vaccines have not been administered at this operation.

Are there outbreaks or occurrences of any of the diseases listed above reported in this operation's area?

Bovine leukosis virus is assumed to occur on virtually all dairies in this area. Sporadic outbreaks of vesicular stomatitis have occurred in the area around this operation.

Mitigations

In this scenario, prevention must focus on insect abatement because vaccination and treatment options for bovine leukosis virus and vesicular stomatitis are not available. The closed-herd status excludes the need to scrutinize the source and disease status of new additions.

Consistent removal of decaying organic matter such as manure, straw, hay, or silage limits breeding sites for stable flies. Introduction of parasitic species of arthropods may also assist in reducing the population of stable flies that feed on cattle. Addition of larvicides to feed may reduce the development of flies. Permethrin dusts, sprays, or pour-ons may be used to control adult stable flies on cattle. The control of black flies is difficult because development occurs in the irrigation ditches adjacent to the operation. Limited options exist to increase the distance of the drylot housing from the irrigation ditches. Control of black flies is limited to the application of animal and premises sprays, which may reduce the density of these vectors.

The sequence of events that transpire between vector acquisition of a pathogen and successful transmission is complex, lengthy, and poorly understood in most cases. The complexity of pathogen maintenance in vectors (overwintering) also adds to the difficulty in developing strategies to prevent disease. Strategies for controlling vectors often are aimed at epidemic or outbreak populations. During such incidences, control is most difficult. Successful prevention of ABDs depends on the integrated or holistic approach, with due consideration given to control of the vector, pathogen and host ecology, and biologic, chemical, and immunologic control mechanisms.

References

[1] APHIS-VS. High Prevalence of BLV in U.S. Dairy Herds. Fort Collins (CO): US Department of Agriculture, Animal and Plant Health Inspection Service, Veterinary Services, Publication No. N228.197, 1997.
[2] Buxton BA, Hinkle NC, Schultz RD. Role of insects in the transmission of bovine leukosis virus: potential for transmission by stable flies, horn flies and tabanids. Am J Vet Res 1985;46:123–6.
[3] Falkner R. Is anaplasmosis spreading in the U.S.? Bovine Veterinarian. 2001;May–June: 24–30.
[4] Fine PEM. Epidemiological principles of vector mediated transmission. In: McKelvey JJ, Eldridge BF, Maramorosch K, editors. Vectors of disease agents: interactions with plants, animals and man. New York: Praeger Publishers; 1981. p. 85.
[5] Gibbs EPJ, Greiner EC. Bluetongue and epizootic hemorraghic disease. In: Monath TP, editor. The arboviruses: epidemiology and ecology, vol. III. Boca Raton (FL): CRC Press; 1988. p. 56.
[6] Harwood RF. Criteria for vector effectiveness. In: McKelvey JJ, Eldridge BF, Maramorosch K, editors. Vectors of disease agents: interactions with plants, animals and man. New York: Praeger Publishers; 1981. p. 5–12.
[7] Hurd HS, McCluskey BJ, Mumford EL. Management factors affecting the risk for vesicular stomatitis in livestock operations in the western United States. J Am Vet Med Assoc 1999;215:1263–8.
[8] Johnson R, Kaneene JB. Bovine leukemia virus, part IV: economic impact and control measures. Comp Cont Educ Prac Vet 1991;11:1727–37.
[9] Kramer WL, Greiner EC, Gibbs EPJ. Seasonal variation in population size, fecundity and parity rates of *Culicoides insignis* (Diptera: Ceraptogonidae) in Florida. USA. J Med Entomol 1985;22:163.

[10] Kuttler KL. Babesiosis. Foreign animal diseases. Richmond (VA): Carter Printing Co.; 1998. p. 81–100.
[11] Maas J. Foothill abortion update. Vet Views November 1995. Available at: www.vetmed. ucdavis.edu.
[12] Martin SW, Meek AH, Willeberg P. Theoretical epidemiology. In: Veterinary epidemiology: principles and methods. Ames (IA): Iowa State University Press; 1987. p. 203–16.
[13] Mead DG, Mare CJ, Ramberg FB. Bite transmission of vesicular stomatitis virus (New Jersey serotype) to laboratory mice by *Simulium vittatum* (Diptera: Simulidae). J Med Entomol 1999;36:410–3.
[14] Radostits OM, Blood DC, Gay CC. Infectious keratitis of cattle. In: Veterinary Medicine, 8th edition. London: Baillere-Tindall; 1994. p. 814.
[15] Rutz DA, Geden CJ, Pitts CW. Pest management recommendations for dairy cattle. Cornell and Penn State Cooperative Extension Publication. College Park (PA): Pennsylvania State University; 2000. p. 1.
[16] Wells SJ. Biosecurity on dairy operations: Hazards and risks. J Dairy Sci 2000;83:2380–6.

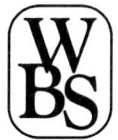

THE VETERINARY
CLINICS
Food Animal
Practice

Vet Clin Food Anim 18 (2002) 115–131

Biosecurity for mammary diseases in dairy cattle

R. Page Dinsmore, DVM

*Department of Clinical Sciences, College of Veterinary Medicine and Biomedical Sciences,
Colorado State University, 300 West Drake Road, Fort Collins, CO 80523, USA*

Biosecurity for control of mammary disease refers to the efforts taken to reduce the introduction of mammary pathogens to a naive herd and reduce the spread of these pathogens between members of the same herd. Biosecurity was recognized as an important means of control of mammary disease long before the term came into common usage. Roberts et al. [44] recommended performing culture tests for all introduced animals to prevent reintroduction of the contagious mastitis pathogen *Streptococcus agalactiae*. Although mastitis is the primary disease discussed in this article, other infectious mammary diseases such as pseudocowpox and herpes mammillitis can appear as devastating outbreaks of teat and udder skin lesions [42,46] that occur after the introduction of cows with active lesions.

Introduction of new animals to dairy herds has become increasingly common, both as a method of replacing culled animals and to increase the number of cattle during herd expansions [35]. Fewer than 10% of herd managers screened introduced cattle by individual culture of milk, and fewer than 25% cultured bulk tank milk from the herds of origin of introduced cattle [35]. Groups of introduced cattle often are assembled from several herds and sale barns without opportunity for pre-sale screening, but veterinarians can help producers avoid substantial losses by insisting that they implement biosecurity measures for control of mastitis.

Mastitis pathogens

Organisms causing mastitis in dairy cattle are generally classified according to their primary source or reservoir. The mammary gland is the reservoir

---

E-mail address: Page.Dinsmore@colostate.edu. (R.P. Dinsmore).

for organisms classified as *contagious mastitis pathogens*, whereas the environment (manure, bedding, corral surfaces) is the source for *environmental mastitis pathogens*. Because of the widespread distribution of environmental mastitis pathogens such as *Escherichia coli* and *Streptococcus uberis*, dairy producers cannot control environmental mastitis by preventing introduction of cows infected with environmental pathogens. Within-herd biosecurity principles for controlling environmental mastitis are not discussed in detail in this article but should include the following: (1) keeping teats and udders clean and dry between milkings, (2) disinfection of teats before milking, and (3) vaccination with *E. coli* core antigen vaccines [47]. On the other hand, control of contagious mastitis requires that infected cattle be prevented from introduction to a herd, and within-herd biosecurity principles to reduce the number of new infections are critically important as well. Each major contagious mastitis pathogen is discussed in the following paragraphs, with particular emphasis on the source and unique features of the control of these pathogens. Measures to limit the spread of all contagious mastitis pathogens are summarized as well.

Streptococcus agalactiae

This organism is the prototypical contagious pathogen. It is an obligate intramammary parasite seldom found outside the mammary gland [31]. In early mastitis literature, it was the most commonly identified agent [34,39, 40,44]. Early surveys found that 40% to 45% of herds had at least one infected cow, and recent Canadian surveys found herd infection rates of 40% (as reviewed by Keefe [28] and Godkin and Leslie [18]). In the author's experience with monthly bulk tank cultures of 84 Colorado herds, the prevalence ranges between 2% and 5% of these herds (R. Page Dinsmore, DVM, unpublished observations, June 2001). In New York State, Wilson and Gonzalez [53] found that 20% of herds in a nonrandomized sample had at least one cow with *S. agalactiae* intramammary infection (IMI).

Procedures for the control and eradication of *S. agalactiae* are well established and successful. Intramammary treatment of infected quarters in either the lactation or the dry period results in greater than 90% cure rates (reviewed by Erskine et al.) [13]. Postmilking teat dipping, dry cow therapy, and the use of separate towels for premilking teat disinfection have been associated with reduced within-herd prevalence of *S. agalactiae* [1].

Progressive dairy producers who are conscious of the benefits of high milk quality do not tolerate the presence of *S. agalactiae* in their herds. Eradication of *S. agalactiae* IMI requires identification of infected cows by milk culture, followed by intramammary antibiotic treatment [44]. This procedure is often carried out as a "blitz" treatment [13,33], in which an entire herd or a substantial portion of it is treated at the same time to effect rapid reduction of the herd prevalence of *S. agalactiae*. Several rounds of culture and treatment may be necessary to eradicate the organism completely. Not all infected cows are identified at each culture; dry cows are not usually sampled, and Dinsmore et al. [11] found that the sensitivity of a single culture for *S. agalactiae* was 95%, indicating that infected cows are classified as negative 5% of the time. Furthermore, treatment is only 87% to 94% effective [51]. During the various rounds of culture and treatment, within-herd biosecurity measures such as postmilking teat dipping and the use of a single towel per cow must be emphasized to prevent the organism from spreading back through the herd.

Eradication of *S. agalactiae* results in substantial expense. Wilson [52] reported losses of $99 and $111 per cow after the introduction, dissemination, and successful eradication of *S. agalactiae*. Culture and treatment to eradicate *S. agalactiae* have been justified by Edmondson [12], however, who found a 41% return on investment 12 months after treatment. Yamagata et al. [54] found a net benefit of treatment of $396 and $237 for cows treated in early and midlactation, respectively. To avoid these significant expenses, between-herd biosecurity practices are clearly warranted and effective. Because the udder is the sole reservoir of infection of *S. agalactiae*, producers with herds that are free of the organism can prevent its introduction by screening herd replacements before they are commingled with an existing herd. Wilson [52] reported costs of $10 per cow in a herd in which a contagious pathogen in introduced cows was identified before it had spread to the remainder of the herd.

Staphylococcus aureus

Although the primary reservoir of *Staphylococcus aureus* is the infected mammary gland, this organism also can be found in many other extramammary sites, such as the nostrils, vagina, and mouth [17]. Prepartum heifers also may be carriers of *Staphylococcus aureus* in the mammary gland [16] and on extramammary sites [43].

With the introduction of antibiotics and the widespread adoption of postmilking teat dipping and dry treatment, herd prevalence of *S. agalactiae* is lower, and *Staphylococcus aureus* has become the most common contagious mastitis pathogen [15]. It has been found that nearly all herds have at least one cow infected with *Staphylococcus aureus*, with herd prevalence ranging from 81% to 94% [8,29,52]. Herd prevalence in 84 Colorado dairies on monthly bulk tank surveillance ranges between 33% and 62% (R. Page Dinsmore, DVM, unpublished observations, June 2001).

Although replacement animals should be screened for *Staphylococcus aureus* before introduction to a herd, it is unlikely that they are the sole source of the organism. Effective control of mastitis due to *Staphylococcus aureus* relies heavily on within-herd biosecurity practices such as postmilking teat dipping and dry cow therapy, for the following reasons:

1. Intramammary antibiotic treatment is often unable to achieve cure rates higher than 50% [13]. Eradication by intramammary treatment is not possible.

2. High US herd prevalence means that purchased replacement cows have a high risk of infection.

3. A single culture for *Staphylococcus aureus* has a sensitivity of 30% to 85%, depending on culture method [10,45], so a single screening culture of replacement cows is likely to fail to identify a significant number of infected cows.

4. Extramammary sources of *Staphylococcus aureus* in cows and heifers represent an ever-present reservoir of the organism, making *Staphylococcus aureus* eradication even less likely.

Dairy producers whose herds have elevated bulk tank somatic cell counts (>300,000/mL) because of high *Staphylococcus aureus* prevalence (>5% of cows) should aim to reduce the number of new infections immediately using the within-herd biosecurity practices summarized previously. The number of existing infections can be reduced as well with culling and treatment, but seldom is eradication possible or cost-effective given the wide variety of sources of *Staphylococcus aureus.* Cure rates of conventional treatment with intramammary antibiotics seldom exceed 20% to 40% [30]. Nickerson [37] recently reviewed several *Staphylococcus aureus* treatment trials and reported that extended therapy with pirlimycin achieved cure rates ranging from 26% to 86%, depending on the herd. Attempts have been made to improve cure rates using extended therapy plus autogenous bacterin immunization [50], but results thus far have not been promising.

Mycoplasma *spp.*

At least 11 species of mycoplasmas are known to cause mastitis in cattle, but most laboratories report that *Mycoplasma bovis* is by far the most common [31], and it is the focus of the following discussion. As a mastitis pathogen, *M. bovis* behaves much like a classical contagious organism. It is extremely infective, in one trial requiring only 70 colony-forming units to initiate infections [3]. Most IMIs originate through the streak canal; fomites include milker's hands, milking equipment, and unsanitary intramammary treatment cannulas [25]. The first described outbreak of mycoplasma mastitis resulted from the use of contaminated penicillin in a multiple-dose intramammary infusion product used to treat 25 of 95 cows with subclinical mastitis [22]. Chronic carriers exist, with intermittent shedding commonly lasting throughout a given lactation and beyond [25]. Although some researchers have shown that certain cows recover spontaneously [9,20], it is not known what proportion of infected animals continues to shed the organism long term.

Some unique features of the biology of *M. bovis* add complexity to the epidemiology of mycoplasma IMI. Although the appearance of mycoplasma mastitis in a naive herd can almost always be traced to the introduction of an infected cow, in rare cases it appears in closed herds [27]. Although it is impossible to prove how an uninfected closed herd develops mycoplasma mastitis, indirect evidence described in the following paragraphs suggests that IMI can occur after respiratory infections in calves and adult cows [20].

Mycoplasmas can be isolated from the nasal cavities of calves in herds without mycoplasma mastitis, although a higher proportion will shed the organism from nasal secretions if fed waste milk from cows with mycoplasma mastitis [5]. Hematogenous dissemination of infection from a variety of primary infection sites (e.g., lung, mammary gland, uterus) has been documented [26], and mastitis has been shown to develop after intravenous inoculation [23]. In the author's experience, calves on a large dairy fed unpasteurized waste milk during a mycoplasma mastitis outbreak developed mycoplasma arthritis and subsequently calved with mycoplasma mastitis (R. Page Dinsmore, DVM, and Meg Cattell, DVM, MS, unpublished observations, 1993). Pasteurization of waste milk on this dairy prevented a recurrence of heifer infections during subsequent outbreaks of mycoplasma mastitis. Cows with clinical mycoplasma mastitis often develop multiple quarter infections. Because the spread to other quarters is not inhibited by the use of quarter milking machines [4], one must assume that spread to other quarters is hematogenous.

Although the preceding theories explaining the origin of mycoplasma mastitis in closed herds must always be kept in mind, most transmission is from cow to cow by infected droplets of milk. Likewise, the appearance of mycoplasma mastitis in a previously uninfected herd is usually attributable to the introduction of an infected cow [25]. Mycoplasma mastitis has been reported from almost every US state and many other regions worldwide [31]. California [31], Florida [7], and New York [19] seem to have more herds infected than other states, but nationwide prevalence studies have not been conducted. There are approximately 150 dairy herds in Colorado, with a total of 89,000 cows; it is estimated that 40% to 50% of these herds have dealt with mycoplasma mastitis, and at least 2000 cows have been sold because of mycoplasma IMI (R. Page Dinsmore, DVM, and Bill Wailes, BS, unpublished observations, 2001). From the standpoint of biosecurity and sourcing of replacement animals, there are no states from which animals can be assumed to be free of mycoplasma mastitis. The most important biosecurity procedure to prevent introduction of mycoplasma mastitis is to screen incoming cattle before they come in contact with the resident herd [31]. Screening programs to monitor the herd must be adopted during expansion to serve as a safeguard in case of accidental introduction of infected cattle.

Screening programs

Individual cow sampling

Culturing individual cow milk samples is the most accurate method of detecting IMIs. For the contagious mastitis pathogens, specificity is 100%

almost by definition, because these pathogens are unlikely to be recovered from milk in the absence of IMI. Sensitivity has been reported as 95% for *S. agalactiae* [11] and 86% for *Staphylococcus aureus* [45]. There are no published reports on the sensitivity of individual cow culture for *Mycoplasma* spp., but some workers estimate the sensitivity to be 24% [53].

Collecting milk samples aseptically from individual cows requires careful attention to technique and can be time consuming and costly on a large scale. To prevent or control an outbreak of contagious mastitis, however, the dairy producer must know the infection status of individual cows. The following sampling strategies are essential biosecurity practices for control of contagious mastitis.

Sample all animals to be introduced to a herd

Ideally, these animals would be sampled before leaving the source farm, and those with contagious mastitis would not be purchased. Larger groups of imported cattle often are assembled from several farms, however, and cattle buyers have historically been reluctant to wait for sampling to be performed. Lactating cows should be sampled immediately on arrival, and dry heifers and cows should be sampled within 2 days of calving. All new animals should be milked last until their culture results are complete.

Sample all lactating cows in the herd

This drastic measure may be necessary under certain specialized circumstances. When deciding whether to sample the entire herd, the factors to consider include the organisms found on screening tests, the herd size and grouping, and the bulk tank cell count history. Whole-herd culture should be performed in the following situations:

- *S. agalactiae* or *Mycoplasma* organisms have been found by a screening test, and the herd is small or cows are maintained in a single group or pen. All animals should be sampled regardless of cell count history. The goal is to identify all infected animals as quickly as possible and treat (*S. agalactiae*) or cull (*Mycoplasma*) infected cattle.
- Any of the three contagious pathogens have been found by a screening test, and the bulk tank cell count has been greater than 500,000 cells/ mL for several months. Cell counts this high for this long indicate that the prevalence of contagious IMI probably exceeds 30%. Little is to be gained from attempting string samples regardless of herd size, because infected cows are likely to be found in all strings.

Sample all cows in particular strings or pens

Herds with multiple pens or strings can often limit the number of cows to be sampled through the use of string samples (see "String Sampling" section). Infected cows are likely to be limited to a smaller number of strings if the contagious pathogens of interest have been discovered during an active expansion, or after monthly or biweekly screening tests have been negative previously, and the bulk tank cell counts are below 400,000/mL.

Sample all heifers and cows as they calve; sample clinical mastitis cases

This technique is important in two situations: (1) during importation of outside animals (replacements or increasing cow numbers), especially if imported animals cannot be sampled before arrival; and (2) during active eradication or segregation during a contagious mastitis outbreak. In either situation, dry cows will not yet have been sampled, and cows are more likely to shed detectable numbers of bacteria at calving [21]. Clinical mastitis is common in cows with new *Mycoplasma* IMIs [26]; culture of these clinical cases serves as an early warning of the spread of this organism and others.

Sample cows with high cell counts

Periodic electronic cell counting (e.g., through Dairy Herd Improvement testing) or herd-wide screening with the California Mastitis Test can be used to identify cows with increased likelihood of IMI. The low sensitivity of cell counts for contagious IMI [53] makes them unsuitable when attempting to eradicate *S. agalactiae* or *Mycoplasma* (tests with high sensitivity are essential for eradication programs). However, monthly or bimonthly culture of cows with high somatic cell counts can be used in addition to fresh cow cultures to identify cows with *Staphylococcus aureus* during situations in which eradication is not the goal.

Bulk tank culture

The bulk tank (BT) is a convenient, accessible source of commingled milk that could theoretically represent all cows in the herd. As such, cultures of BT milk have been performed since the late 1960s to screen for contagious mastitis pathogens while avoiding the expense of culturing all individual cows in a herd [14,29]. In the past decade, researchers have attempted to describe the properties of BT culture as a screening test for contagious mastitis pathogens. The sensitivity of a single BT culture for *S. agalactiae* IMI has been reported as 20.5% [18], 35.3% [2], and 77% [53]. For *Staphylococcus aureus*, the reported sensitivities were 9.2%, 42.2%, and 58% [2,18,53]. Wilson and Gonzalez [53] found the sensitivity of BT culture for *Mycoplasma* IMI to be 33%. Various researchers have improved the sensitivity of BT culture for contagious IMI by using selective media [14,32,41] and performing serial sampling over several days (reviewed by Godkin and Leslie) [18]. Farnsworth [14] now recommends that for optimal sensitivity, samples from 4 days should be collected and pooled, and sampling should be conducted on a monthly or bimonthly basis depending on herd size. Samples then should be plated on TKT-FC media for selection of streptococci; KLMB media to distinguish staphylococci; MacConkey's media for coliform counts; and a selective mycoplasma medium such as Hayflick's. Despite these techniques, some important contagious IMIs will fail to be detected in large herds, however. It is not known precisely how herd size and infection prevalence influence the sensitivity of BT culture, but it is suggested (Greg Goodell, DVM, personal communication, June 2001) that practitioners treating herds with more than 300 milking cows may miss the introduction of contagious pathogens even under the best BT sampling and culture techniques, and string sampling should be adopted.

String sampling

In an attempt to increase the sensitivity of group culturing without resorting to whole-herd sampling, collection of commingled milk from strings or pens of cows seems to be gaining in popularity in the author's experience and is becoming widely adopted in large herds in the West. In general, *string sampling* refers to the collection of a "drip" sample of milk during milking of a particular pen of cows. As successive strings or pens of cows enter the parlor, new collection vials are filled and labeled. The obvious advantage of string sampling over BT sampling is the size of the group: on all but the largest herds, pens typically hold 100 to 250 cows. No research has been conducted to evaluate the sensitivity of string sampling, but studies on BT culturing in small herds should be applicable. Furthermore, string sampling allows the dairy producer to focus on a particular high-risk group, again without culturing each individual. For instance, some dairies leave all cows in a "fresh" pen for the first 7 to 14 days after calving. Weekly string sampling of this pen will screen every cow in the herd for a year. Likewise, the sick pen represents an area likely to contain cows shedding contagious pathogens such as *Mycoplasma*. Because milk from sick-pen cows is withheld from the BT, contagious IMI in sick-pen cows would fail to be detected in a BT culture.

It is worthwhile to discuss the technical details involved in string sample collection. If a single pen is to be sampled, and that pen happens to be milked into an empty tank, the simplest solution is to collect a BT sample after the last cow from that pen has been milked. It should be obvious, however, that to collect separate samples from all pens in the herd, serial BT samples would not be appropriate: if the first pen contained infected cows, all subsequent serial samples also would be culture positive. String samples should be collected from the positive pressure side of the milking system, from a section of milk transfer pipe between the milk transfer pump and the BT (Fig. 1). An ideal collection system is shown in Figs. 2A and B, in which a sample valve is welded into a replaceable section of milk transfer line. A less elegant collection system is shown in Fig. 3: a clamp on a gasketed joint in the milk line is loosened to allow milk to drip each time the transfer pump is activated. Other modifications include the use of a Vacutainer needle (Becton-Dickson) inserted through the gasket of a similar joint in the milk line (Mark Wustenberg, DVM, personal communication, March 2000) or a

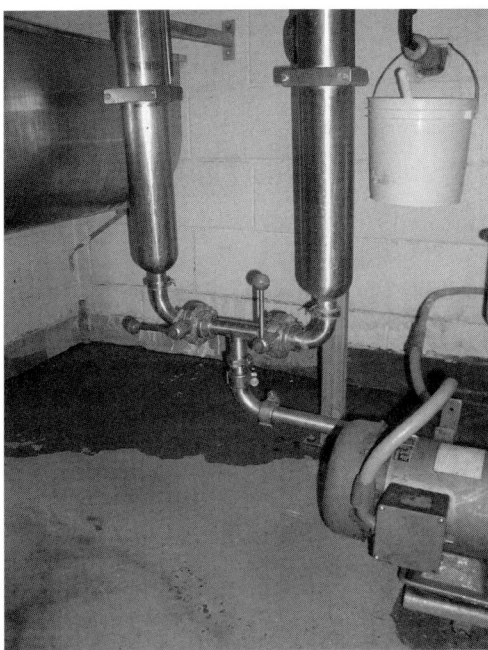

Fig. 1. Potential site for string sampling of milk to screen for contagious mastitis pathogens. Sample should be collected from the milk line, between the milk transfer pump (*lower right*) and bulk tank.

special diaphragm clamped onto a T connection (Scott Meyer, BS, personal communication, March 2000).

Based on the author's experience with dairy expansions and udder health in Colorado, it has become painfully obvious that today's expanding herds must assume that it is not a matter of "if" contagious mastitis will appear but "when." A comprehensive program or standard operating procedure must be designed and implemented before new cows are introduced. All new cows must be cultured as soon as possible after arrival, but the screening program must assume that some infected cows will not be identified before other cows are infected. To identify the occurrence of contagious mastitis in the resident herd before a full-blown outbreak occurs, BT and string samples must be cultured on a weekly basis as well as samples from all fresh cows and cows with clinical mastitis. Flow charts for mammary disease biosecurity in both closed and open herds are provided (Figs. 4 and 5).

Control of contagious mastitis

In addition to the control procedures specific to individual pathogens described previously, some general principles of contagious mastitis control must be reviewed. All of these principles serve to reduce the number of new infections in an existing herd [15].

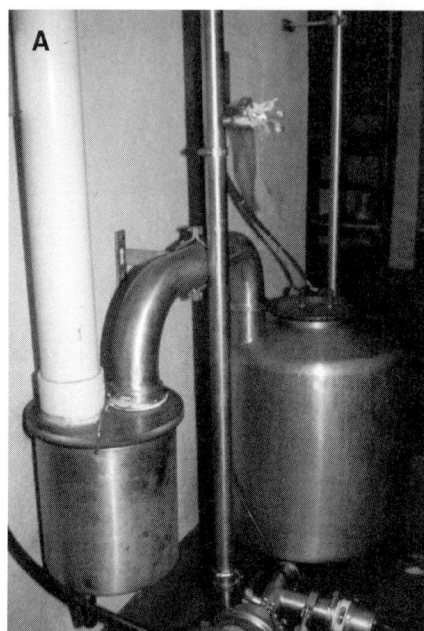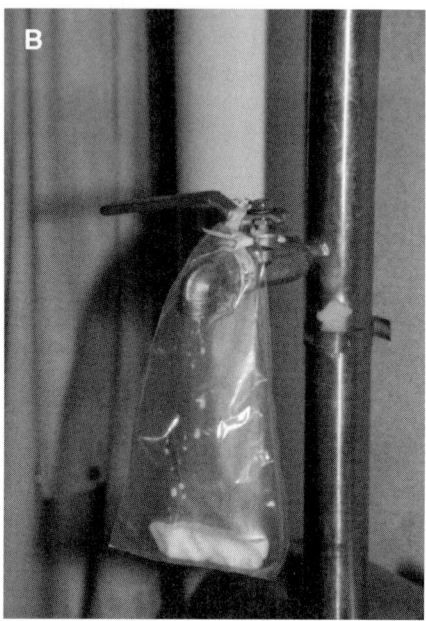

Fig. 2. (A) string sample collection valve. Note location downstream from milk transfer pump (*bottom center*). (B) close-up view of valve.

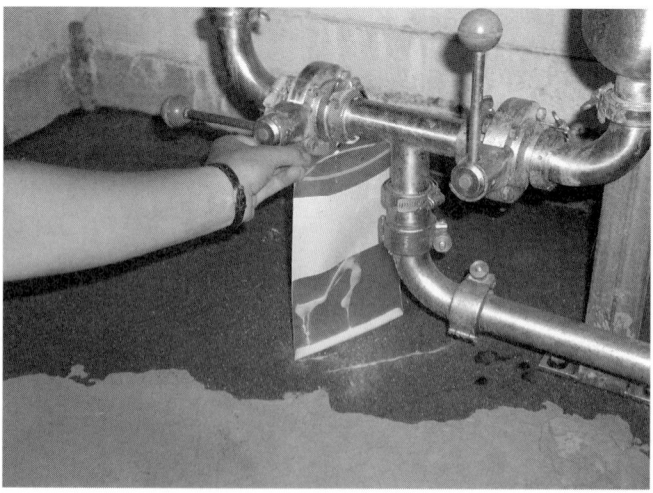

Fig. 3. String sample collection. Clamp has been loosened to allow milk to drip into collection bag as milk transfer pump is activated.

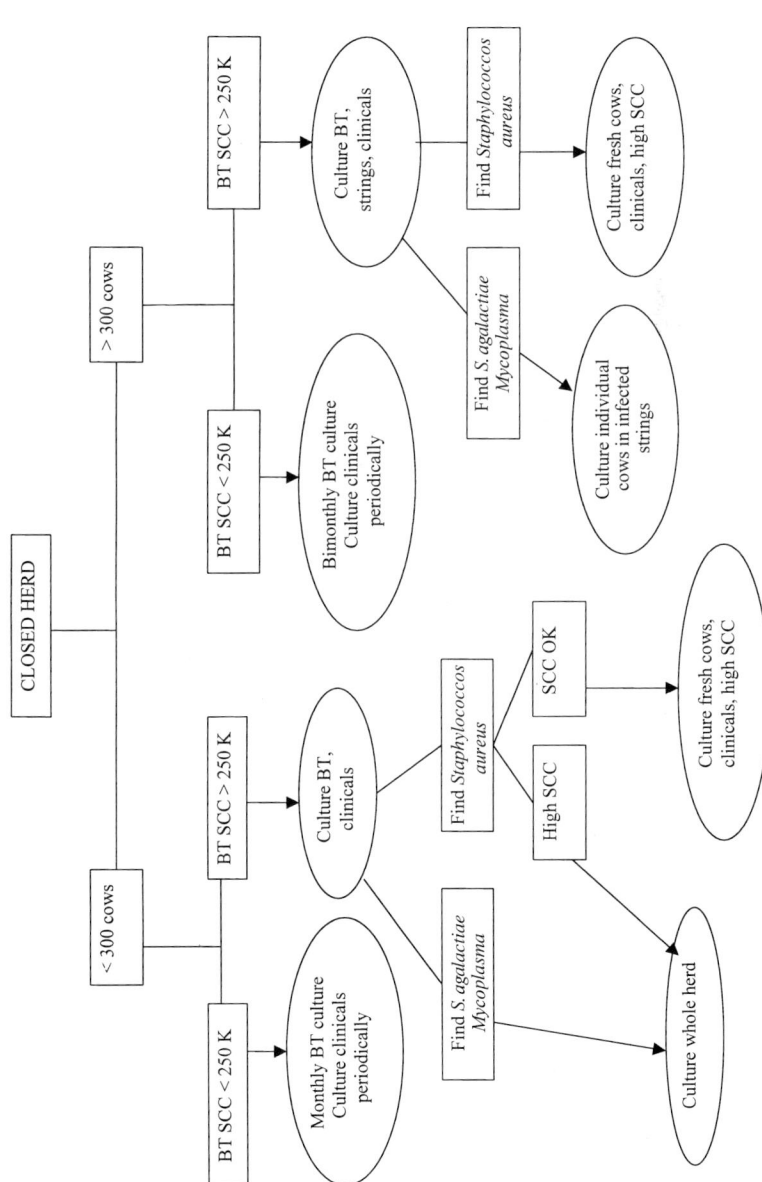

Fig. 4. Mammary disease biosecurity for closed herds. BT = bulk tank; SCC = somatic cell count.

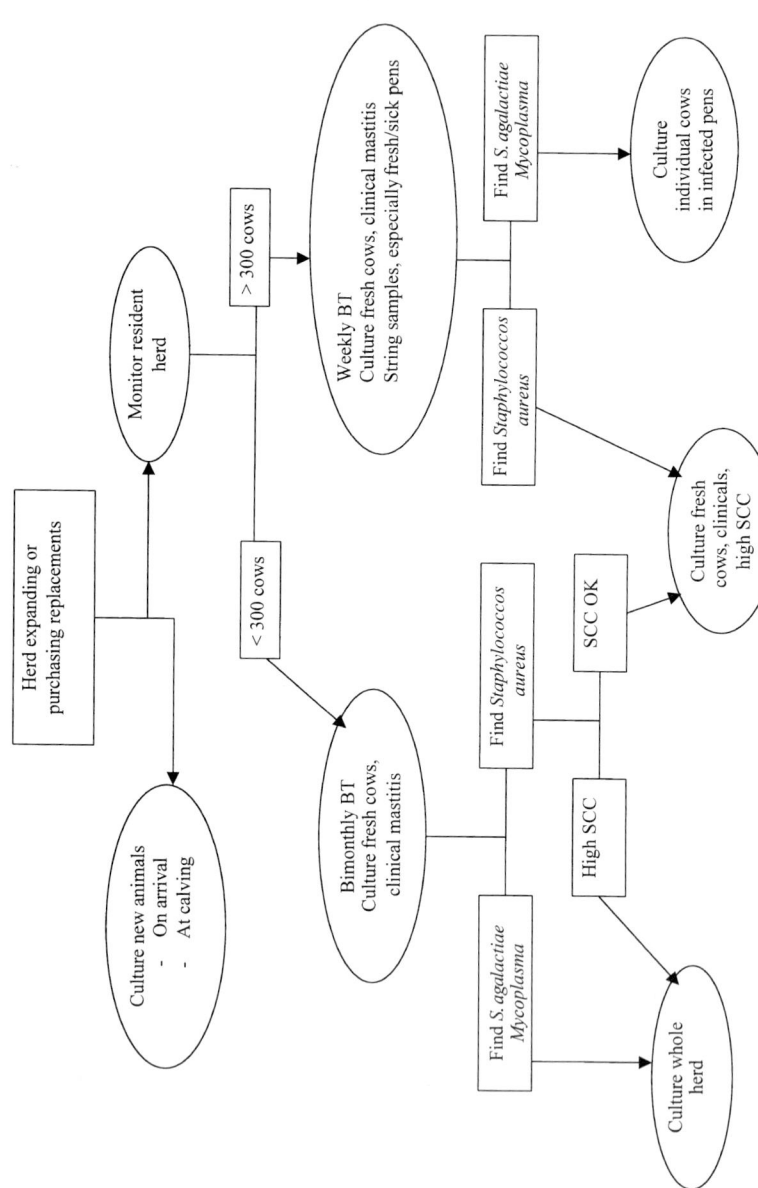

Fig. 5. Mammary disease biosecurity for expansion of open herds. BT = bulk tank; SCC = somatic cell count.

Preparation of the cow for milking

The teats of all cows should be disinfected before attachment of milking machines to reduce the risk of environmental mastitis infections; however, teat ends and milkers' hands also can become contaminated with milk from cows infected with contagious mastitis pathogens. To reduce the transfer of these bacteria from cow to cow, milkers should wear latex or nitrile gloves, apply a disinfectant such as a premilking teat dip to all teats, and use single-service paper or cloth towels to remove disinfectant and any residual manure or dirt.

Contribution of milking equipment to spread of contagious mastitis

It is estimated that approximately 6% of mastitis infections are caused by milking equipment [49]. There are three ways in which milking equipment can contribute to new contagious IMI rates [24]. First, the equipment can cause direct injury to teat ends because of excessive teat-end vacuum, excess machine on-time, or inadequate pulsation. Injury to teat ends greatly increases the susceptibility of the quarter to IMI caused by contagious pathogens, especially *S. aureus*. The claw vacuum should not exceed 14.5 inches of Hg (49.5 kPa) and should range between 11 and 12 in Hg.

A second method by which milking equipment can contribute to new contagious IMI is by carrying pathogens from one cow to the next, or from one infected quarter to a noninfected quarter of the same cow. Many attempts have been made to document the benefits of disinfecting milking units between cows using automated backflush systems. Although backflush systems have been shown to reduce the numbers of bacteria on milking equipment dramatically, reductions of contagious pathogen IMI have been modest at best [48]. To reduce the transfer of contagious pathogens effectively, chronically infected cows should be segregated from the rest of the herd and milked last.

Intramammary infection can be caused by reverse pressures or impacts during milking [24]. These events are caused by the sudden introduction of air into one or more liners during milking as the result of liner slips or removal of units under vacuum. Liner slips occur most often toward the end of milking. Modern lightweight claws and narrow bore liners have reduced liner slips, but it is unlikely that they will ever be eliminated given the wide variety of teat shapes and milking system configurations. Therefore, milkers should be trained to recognize and correct liner slips as soon as possible. Vacuum must be shut off before unit removal, either with a manual valve or automatic detachment systems [24].

Postmilking teat disinfection

Application of a germicidal solution immediately after milking is the single most effective practice for the prevention of contagious IMI [38]. An excellent review of publications on the efficacy of teat disinfections was published by the National Mastitis Council [36]. Iodine is by far the most common disinfectant; other common disinfectants include chlorhexidine, linear dodecyl benzene sulfonic acid, lauryl sulfate, and sodium chlorite/lactic acid. The traditional method of teat dip application is the cup, allowing near-total immersion of the teat in the disinfectant. Concern has been expressed regarding contamination of teat dip containers with environmental bacteria. Teat spray systems have been widely adopted in large parlors for convenience and speed. Such systems are implicated frequently as contributing to the spread of contagious mastitis [7]; because rapid through-put is so important in large dairies, milkers tend not to cover all teats with dip when using spray systems. Only one small recent study has compared spraying and dipping [6]; in a natural exposure trial, total IMIs were almost identical. Dipped cows had four *Staphylococcus aureus* IMIs versus 15 for sprayed cows, however. Had the trial been performed in a large rapid-throughput parlor, one might speculate that the *Staphylococcus aureus* IMI difference would be even greater, favoring dip cup application versus spray application.

Dry treatment

Treatment of all quarters of all cows at dryoff is a standard practice on US dairy farms. This procedure may be more effective than lactation treatment at eliminating infections due to streptococci and staphylococci, and dry treatment reduces the number of new infections that develop at the onset of the dry period (reviewed by Erskine et al.) [13].

Summary

As US dairies grow ever larger and obtain replacement animals from a wide geographical area, biosecurity will loom ever more important as a means of controlling mammary disease. To prevent costly outbreaks of contagious mastitis, introduced animals must be screened for contagious IMI before the resident herd is exposed to them. Screening programs must be instituted to detect the appearance of contagious IMI as soon as possible after introduction has occurred. Most importantly, 40 years of knowledge regarding the on-farm control of contagious mastitis (now known as within-herd biosecurity) must be dusted off and implemented with renewed vigor to prevent the rampant spread of contagious mastitis.

References

[1] Bartlett PC, Miller GY, Lance SE, et al. Managerial risk factors of intramammary infection with *Streptococcus agalactiae* in dairy herds in Ohio. Am J Vet Res 1992;53: 1715–20.

[2] Bartlett PC, Miller GY, Lance SE, et al. Use of bulk tank and milk filter cultures in screening for *Streptococcus agalactiae* and coagulase-positive staphylococci. J Food Protect 1991;54:848–51.

[3] Bennett RH, Jasper DE. Bovine mycoplasmal mastitis from intramammary inoculations of small numbers of *Mycoplasma bovis*: local and systemic antibody response. Am J Vet Res 1980;41:889–92.

[4] Bennett RH, Jasper DE. Bovine mycoplasmal mastitis from intramammary inoculations of small numbers of *Mycoplasma bovis*: I. microbiology and pathology. Vet Microbiol 1977–1978;2:341–55.

[5] Bennett RH, Jasper DE. Nasal prevalence of *Mycoplasma bovis* and IHA titers in young dairy animals. Cornell Vet 1977;67:361–73.

[6] Boddie RL, Nickerson SC, Doyle M. Comparison of postmilking teat dipping with teat spraying under natural exposure conditions. In: Proceedings of the 37th Annual Meeting of the National Mastitis Council; 1998. p. 263–4.

[7] Bray DR, Shearer JK, Donovan GA, et al. Approaches to achieving and maintaining a herd free of mycoplasma mastitis. In: Proceedings of the 36th Annual Meeting of the National Mastitis Council, Albuquerque (NM); 1997. p. 132–7.

[8] Britten AM, Emerson T. A bulk tank culturing program for monitoring milk quality and udder health. In: Proceedings of the 35th Annual Meeting of the National Mastitis Council, Nashville (TN); 1996. p. 149–50.

[9] Brown MB, Shearer JK, Elvinger F. Mycoplasmal mastitis in a dairy herd. J Am Vet Med Assoc 1990;196:1097–101.

[10] Buelow K, Nordlund K. Factors affecting sensitivity and specificity of microbiological culture for *Staphylococcus aureus*. In: Proceedings of the 38th Annual Meeting of the National Mastitis Council, Arlington (VA); 1999. p. 68–75.

[11] Dinsmore PR, English PB, Gonzalez RN, et al. Evaluation of methods for the diagnosis of *Streptococcus agalactiae* intramammary infections in dairy cattle. J Dairy Sci 1991;74: 1521–6.

[12] Edmondson PW. An economic justification of "blitz" therapy to eradicate *Streptococcus agalactiae* from a dairy herd. Vet Rec 1989;125:591–3.

[13] Erskine RJ, Kirk JH, Tyler JW, et al. Advances in the therapy for mastitis. Vet Clin North Am 1993;9:499–517.

[14] Farnsworth RJ. Microbiologic examination of bulk tank milk. Vet Clin North Am Large Anim Pract 1993;9:469–74.

[15] Fox LK, Gay JM. Contagious mastitis. Vet Clin North Am Large Anim Pract 1993;9:475–87.

[16] Fox LK, Chester ST, Hallberg JW, et al. Survey of intramammary infections in dairy heifers at breeding age and first parturition. J Dairy Sci 1995;78:1619–28.

[17] Fox LK, Middleton JR, Biosecurity and *Staphylococcus aureus* mastitis: do replacement and expansion cattle pose a risk? In: Proceedings of the Regional Meeting of the National Mastitis Council, Bellevue (WA); 1998. p. 1–8.

[18] Godkin MA, Leslie KE. Culture of bulk tank milk as a mastitis screening test: a brief review. Can Vet J 1993;34:601–5.

[19] Gonzalez RN, Sears PM. Occurrence of bovine mycoplasmal mastitis in herds and cows in the state of New York. In: Proceedings of the 34th Annual Meeting of the National Mastitis Council, Fort Worth (TX); 1995. p. 128–9.

[20] Gonzalez RN, Jayarao BM, Oliver SP, et al. Pneumonia, arthritis and mastitis in dairy cows due to *Mycoplasma bovis*. In: Proceedings of the 32nd Annual Meeting of the National Mastitis Council, Kansas City (MO); 1993. p. 178–86.

[21] Gonzalez RN, Sears PM, Wilson DJ, et al. Can we manage *Mycoplasma bovis* infected herds without intensive culling? In: Proceedings of the 33rd Annual Meeting of the National Mastitis Council, Orlando (FL); 1994. p. 360–1.

[22] Hale HH, Helmboldt CF, Plastridge WN, et al. Bovine mastitis caused by a *Mycoplasma* species. Cornell Vet 1962;52:582–91.

[23] Jain NC, Jasper DE, Dellinger JD. Experimental bovine mastitis due to *Mycoplasma*. Cornell Vet 1969;59:10–28.

[24] Jarrett JA. Mechanical milking and its relationship to mastitis. Vet Clin North Am Large Anim Pract 1984;6:349–60.

[25] Jasper DE. Bovine mycoplasmal mastitis. J Am Vet Med Assoc 1979;175:1072–4.

[26] Jasper DE. Mycoplasma and mycoplasma mastitis. J Am Vet Med Assoc 1977;170:1167–72.

[27] Jasper DE. The role of *Mycoplasma* in bovine mastitis. J Am Vet Med Assoc 1982;181:158–62.

[28] Keefe GP. *Streptococcus agalactiae* mastitis: a review. Can Vet J 1997;38:429–37.

[29] Kelton D, Alves D, Smart N, et al. Bulk tank culture for major contagious mastitis pathogens: lessons from the sentinel herds. In: Proceedings of the 38th Annual Meeting of the National Mastitis Council, Arlington (VA); 1999. p. 144–5.

[30] Kirk JH. Diagnosis and treatment of difficult mastitis cases. Agri-Practice 1991;12:5–8.

[31] Kirk JH, Lauerman LH. *Mycoplasma* mastitis in dairy cows. Compend Contin Educ Pract Vet 1994;16:541–51.

[32] Ollis GW, Rawluk SA, Schoonderwoerd M, et al. Detection of *Staphylococcus aureus* in bulk tank milk using modified Baird-Parker culture media. Can Vet J 1995;36:619–23.

[33] McDonald JS. Streptococcal and staphylococcal mastitis. Vet Clin North Am Large Anim Pract 1984;6:269–85.

[34] Murphy JM. Mastitis—the struggle for understanding. J Dairy Sci 1956;39:1768–73.

[35] National Animal Health Monitoring System. Dairy '96, part 1: reference of 1996 dairy management. Fort Collins (CO): USDA:APHIS:VS, CEAH, National Animal Health Monitoring System, 1996.

[36] National Mastitis Council. Summary of peer-reviewed publications on efficacy of premilking and postmilking teat disinfectants published since 1980. In: Proceedings of the 40th Annual Meeting of the National Mastitis Council, Madison (WI); 2001. p. 271–83.

[37] Nickerson SC. Role of vaccination and treatment programs. In: Proceedings of the 38th Annual Meeting of the National Mastitis Council, Arlington (VA); 1999. p. 76–85.

[38] Pankey JW. Postmilking teat antisepsis. Vet Clin North Am Large Anim Pract 1984;6:335–48.

[39] Peterson EH, Hastings EG, Hadley FB. The pathology of nonspecific mastitis and consideration of possible etiological agents. Cornell Vet 1938;28:307–24.

[40] Plastridge WN. Bovine mastitis: a review. J Dairy Sci 1958;41:1141–81.

[41] Postle DS. Evaluation of a selective medium for screening bulk milk samples for *Streptococcus agalactiae*. Am J Vet Res 1968;29:669–78.

[42] Rebhun WC. Diseases of the teats and udder. In: Rebhun WB, editor. Diseases of dairy cattle. Media (PA): Williams & Wilkins; 1995. p. 275–6.

[43] Roberson JR, Fox LK, Hancock DD, et al. Sources of intramammary infections from *Staphylococcus aureus* in dairy heifers at first parturition. J Dairy Sci 1998;81:687–93.

[44] Roberts SJ, Hodges HC, Fincher MG, et al. Studies of the *Streptococcus agalactiae* form of mastitis in dairy cattle. J Am Vet Med Assoc 1963;143:1193–201.

[45] Sears PM, Smith BS, English PB, et al. Shedding pattern of *Staphylococcus aureus* from bovine intramammary infections. J Dairy Sci 1990;73:2785–9.

[46] Sieber RL, Farnsworth RJ. Differential diagnosis of bovine teat lesions. Vet Clin North Am Large Anim Pract 1984;6:313–21.

[47] Smith KL, Hogan JS. Environmental mastitis. Vet Clin North Am Food Anim Pract 1993;9:489–98.

[48] Smith TW, Eberhart RJ, Spencer SB, et al. Effect of automatic backflushing on number of new intramammary infections, bacteria on teat cup liners, and milk iodine. J Dairy Sci 1985;68:424–35.

[49] Spencer SB. Recent research and developments in machine milking: a review. J Dairy Sci 1989;72:1907–17.

[50] Timms L, Kirkpatrick M, Sears PM. Field trial evaluation of extended pirlimycin therapy with or without vaccination for *Staphylococcus aureus* mastitis. In: Proceedings of the 39th Annual Meeting of the National Mastitis Council, Atlanta (GA); 2000. p. 201–2.

[51] Weaver LD, Galland J, Martin PAJ, et al. Treatment of *Streptococcus agalactiae* mastitis in dairy cows: comparative efficacies of two antibiotic preparations and factors associated with successful treatment. J Am Vet Med Assoc 1986;189:666–9.

[52] Wilson DJ. Mastitis biosecurity: lessons from expansion in New York. In: Proceedings of the Regional Meeting of the National Mastitis Council, Waterloo, Ontario; 1999. p. 10–17.

[53] Wilson DJ, Gonzalez RN. Evaluation of milk culture, SCC, and CMT for screening herd additions. In: Proceedings of the 36th Annual Meeting of the National Mastitis Council, Albuquerque (NM); 1997. p. 127–31.

[54] Yamagata M, Goodger WJ, Weaver LD, et al. The economic benefit of treating subclinical *Streptococcus agalactiae* mastitis in lactating cows. J Am Vet Med Assoc 1987;191: 1556–61.

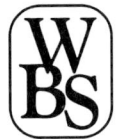

THE VETERINARY
CLINICS
Food Animal
Practice

Vet Clin Food Anim 18 (2002) 133–155

Biosecurity of veterinary practices

Paul S. Morley, DVM, PhD

Veterinary Teaching Hospital, Colorado State University, Fort Collins, CO 80523, USA

Biosecurity refers to all hygienic practices designed to prevent occurrences of infectious diseases. This includes preventing introduction of infectious agents, controlling their spread within populations or facilities, and containment or disinfection of infectious materials. Biosecurity is affected tremendously by the ecology of animal and human populations, the biologic nature of infectious agents, and by management actions that affect interactions between host and agent. This aspect of husbandry has gained increasing attention in the past few years from producers and veterinarians. Globalization of the economy has increased pressures to control and regionally eradicate infectious diseases to preserve marketability of livestock and animal products. At the same time, trends in livestock production are toward larger, more intensive production units that have undoubtedly increased the risk of introduction and transmission of infectious agents. Veterinarians and hospital facilities likely play a role in this increased risk of disease transmission, conflicting with desires to make veterinarians an integral part of the production team. The litigious nature of modern business environments adds another stimulus for improved biosecurity, as do political and social pressures for increased food safety.

Nosocomial infections in veterinary hospitals are not solely a patient-care concern; the spread of infectious agents also can significantly affect normal hospital operations, revenue, client confidence, public image, and the morale of hospital personnel. In some cases nosocomial agents are also zoonotic. In 1996, Colorado State University's Veterinary Teaching Hospital (CSU-VTH) experienced an outbreak of *Salmonella infantis* in their large animal facility [21]. This outbreak involved a total of 59 animals, primarily horses, and the death of three animals was attributed to complications from *S. Infantis* infection. The large animal hospital was temporarily closed twice because of this epidemic, which resulted in an estimated $300,000 in lost revenues in addition to $250,000 required for facility renovation. These financial losses do not account for intangible losses such as diminished client

E-mail address: paul.morley@colostate.edu (P.S. Morley)

confidence, morale problems among hospital personnel, and lost learning opportunities for students. Fortunately this *Salmonella* outbreak at CSU did not result in identifiable human illness or infection, but exposure to a variety of zoonotic agents has been documented at other times in association with care of veterinary patients [5,11,14,19]

This type of outbreak is not unusual at large veterinary facilities. According to a 1997 survey of veterinary teaching hospitals in the United States, 12 of 18 veterinary schools that responded reported 18 outbreaks of nosocomial disease between 1985 and 1996 (Dr. A.W. Nelson, DVM, PhD, personal communication, Fort Collins, CO, 2000). Seventy-eight percent of outbreaks were attributed to *Salmonella*. High caseload was cited by eight respondents as being a significant contributor to the risk of nosocomial disease spread. Forty-three percent (n = 6) of *Salmonella*-associated outbreaks resulted in hospital closure, and estimated costs per outbreak ranged from approximately $10,000 to $550,000. At the time of this survey, only half of the respondents had active infection control committees, and only three employed a person responsible for infection control at the hospital.

Although most of the preceding information comes from events at large veterinary teaching hospitals, the same effects can and do occur in smaller, private veterinary practices. This article discusses the need for biosecurity programs in veterinary practices and describes a practical approach for developing biosecurity practices that are tailored to individual facilities.

Why is biosecurity important for veterinary practices?

Hospitalization of sick animals tremendously increases their risk of acquiring infections because it congregates animals that are most likely to be shedding infectious agents with animals that often have enhanced susceptibility. Removing livestock from their home environment, transporting them, and confining them in proximity to unfamiliar animals also likely affects inherent susceptibility to infection because of stress. Ambulatory practices are not immune to risks associated with infectious diseases. Clothing, equipment, and vehicles can easily become contaminated with infectious agents, and veterinarians can become vectors for disease transmission unwittingly as they move among animal populations.

To provide the best veterinary care possible, veterinarians have an underlying responsibility to minimize the risk of additional harm that might unintentionally befall an animal because of their interventions. This responsibility includes minimizing the risk of exposing patients to infectious agents. It is therefore incumbent on veterinarians to manage the risk of nosocomial infections actively.

In evaluating the benefits of formal biosecurity programs, it is perhaps useful to consider an example of such a program, the biosecurity program at CSU-VTH. The biosecurity program at CSU-VTH is a proactive prevention program designed to identify hazards before they become problematic to personnel, patients, or the normal operation of the hospital. In the wake of the 1996 *Salmonella* outbreak at CSU-VTH, this rigorous biosecurity program was formalized in an effort to minimize the risk of nosocomial and zoonotic infections. A faculty position was created to oversee this program, and ongoing funding was committed for a house officer to work and train in this area.

The four goals of the CSU-VTH biosecurity program are as follows: (1) to reduce the risk of zoonotic disease and promote public health among hospital personnel and clients, (2) to provide an environment in which patient care is optimized by minimizing the threat of nosocomial infections, (3) to promote the development of lifelong skills in public health and biosecurity among hospital personnel, and (4) to protect CSU-VTH from financial loss and litigation. This program works to minimize the risk of myriad nosocomial and zoonotic health problems. Some of these diseases are important to producers, although they might be considered more of a nuisance than medically important (e.g., contagious respiratory diseases such as influenza and kennel cough, infestations with fleas and lice). Some diseases targeted by this program are potentially life-threatening nosocomial infections such as salmonellosis, wound infections, and septicemias. Some have considerable regulatory importance such as vesicular stomatitis or foot-and-mouth disease. Other diseases are important to the biosecurity program because they are important zoonotic diseases such as cryptosporidiosis, rabies, and plague (*Yersinia pestis* infection). In the current international political climate, CSU-VTH also has increased its vigilance to prevent intentional introduction of infectious agents at the facility and to detect unusual illness among animals as they are presented by clients.

The author's experiences with biosecurity concerns since the inception of the program suggest that more rigorous biosecurity precautions are becoming a necessary part of standard-of-care expectations. The author and his colleagues at CSU-VTH have received numerous inquiries from veterinarians and animal owners regarding control and prevention of nosocomial infections. We have found that our biosecurity program is an important aid to patient and facility management at CSU-VTH. Personal communications with colleagues throughout the United States and Canada indicate that biosecurity programs are being developed at referral centers that are similar to or modeled after the CSU-VTH biosecurity program. Many of these programs have been developed at private and public facilities in response to experiences that are similar to the 1996 *Salmonella* epidemic at CSU as described previously. We also have been contacted by veterinarians in private practice and animal owners because of pending legal action related to nosocomial disease.

The importance of surveillance

When discussing the use of biosecurity programs in veterinary practices, the author is told by some veterinarians that they do not need additional precautions because they do not have a problem; however, further discussion often reveals that they do not actually know if nosocomial transmission is occurring because they do not look for it. There is considerable wisdom in the adage, "You cannot manage what is not measured."

Surveillance is an important tool for management of any operation, including veterinary practices. Managers must have feedback regarding the status of the system so that corrective action can be taken when necessary. In fact, monitoring programs provide the foundation for any planned veterinary service in food animal production [18], and there are multiple benefits to using such programs. Monitoring programs provide information regarding the current status of the operation. They can help pinpoint problem areas that should be targeted for additional investigation or corrective action, which assists in making disease prevention efforts efficient and economical by identifying where resources are needed most. Regular review of data gathered from monitoring programs stimulates re-evaluation of disease prevention strategies. Monitoring programs can provide early warning for veterinarians and producers regarding problems that threaten productivity before these problems become large and unmanageable.

Should your practice use a formal biosecurity program?

Beyond realizing the importance of infection control and biosecurity, there is a critical need to evaluate whether a specific veterinary practice needs to enact a *formal* biosecurity program, and how much rigor is appropriate. Practicing veterinarians routinely perform actions that decrease the risk of disease transmission (e.g., sterilizing surgical instruments, washing hands and boots); however, the sum of these individual actions does not necessarily equate with enacting a systematized biosecurity program. The latter implies that a thoughtful, logical approach is being used to systematically reduce the risk of transmitting infectious agents in the process of delivering veterinary care. These actions may target specific agents and diseases, or they may be more generally intended to improve hygiene and thereby reduce contamination for a number of agents.

Determining if a formal biosecurity program should be enacted or if existing actions need to be enhanced requires careful consideration of disease risks and an equally thoughtful consideration of the level of risk aversion that is appropriate for a practice. No "one-size-fits-all" program can be transferred from one practice to another. What is practical and reasonable for some veterinarians in their practice situation may be untenable and unreasonable for others. A useful exercise is to make a comprehensive list of all infectious agents that can be transmitted among patients in the practice. Zoonotic diseases also should be considered in this list. Once this list is complete, each disease should be categorized according to the overall risk that it poses for the practice. Many factors influence the relative importance of diseases to a specific practice. These factors include biologic characteristics of the agents (i.e., contagiousness, pathogenicity, and the ability of an agent to persist in the environment), the characteristics of the patient population (i.e., immune versus susceptible), the value of patients in one's care, the health concerns of veterinary personnel and clients regarding zoonotic agents, and the risk of damage to one's practice if nosocomial infections were to occur (e.g., lost revenue, costs for cleaning a contaminated facility, damaged professional reputation, and the potential for legal action). Another aspect to consider is that there is considerable variability in the pathogenicity and medical importance among different strains of various agents. An interesting common feature of many documented and undocumented outbreaks of nosocomial bacterial infections is that the organisms are often resistant to a large number of important antimicrobial drugs [1,13,15,20,21] . It is not clear if multidrug-resistant bacteria are more likely to become resident in a hospital environment, or if they are more likely to be noticed than are nosocomial infections that can be treated with standard antibiotic regimens. Regardless, it can be difficult to effectively treat multiple animals infected with resistant bacteria, just as it is tremendously difficult to explain to several clients that these infections were unforeseen and not preventable.

After ordering hazards identified in this process according to their relative importance, precautions that are currently being taken to prevent introduction or the spread of each agent should be cataloged. An assessment of current operating procedures that might increase the risk of disease transmission also should be made.

It should be recognized that failure to take necessary precautions and breakdowns in performance are not the only causes of biosecurity problems. Experience at CSU-VTH suggests that a heightened desire to provide optimal care for individual patients and the needs of clients can also sometimes impair the ability of veterinarians and support personnel to appropriately gauge the immediate importance of their actions relative to biosecurity for the larger population or the practice. In fact, actions taken to provide every possible benefit for the individual can sometimes be directly contrary to the greater good of other patients and the practice. For example, given the stresses produced by hospitalizing some large animal patients in unfamiliar enclosed environments, it might be beneficial to house livestock outdoors in dirt- or grass-based enclosures for recuperation. A single animal shedding an environmentally persistent agent such as *Salmonella*, however, can extensively contaminate these environments, which are impossible to disinfect completely. The risk of nosocomial disease also can be inadvertently increased for individual patients when rigorous management practices are used, as is the case regarding frequent physical contact with patients. More frequent evaluation and treatment may be thought to ensure an animal's well-being but also increase the potential for inadvertent transmission of infectious agents, particularly if there are animals in a facility with a high risk of shedding infectious agents.

This risk-assessment process should then lead to an appraisal of whether current operating procedures are sufficient to protect one's patients and practice, considering the relative importance of each agent or whether there is a mismatch between risk assessment and the level of risk aversion. It is critical in this process to consider realistically whether current biosecurity precautions are followed routinely. In this regard, it should be realized that a manager's impression of what *should* be done does not always coincide with the procedures *actually* used by personnel. If actions do not appear to match the potential risks and the level of risk aversion, a more rigorous formalized program seems appropriate. At minimum, this should provide a basis for evaluation of procedural options to determine whether they can reasonably be incorporated to assist management of the veterinary practice.

Designing a tailored biosecurity program

An effective biosecurity program must be tailored to the needs and limitations of each individual operation. As discussed previously, it is not possible to take a biosecurity program designed for one practice and simply apply it in another operation without modification. There are systematic approaches that can be used to assist in the design of disease management programs, however. Applying the Hazard Analysis and Critical Control Point (HACCP) concepts is one such systematic approach that the author has found quite useful in a variety of situations. The HACCP concepts were originally developed to manage potential hazards to food production industries, and more recently were incorporated into regulations used by the US Department of Agriculture, Food Safety Inspection Service to minimize introduction of pathogens into the US food supply [23]. This systematic approach for identifying and managing operation hazards is ideally suited for guiding infectious disease control efforts in operations such as that of CSU-VTH or other veterinary practices.

The HACCP approach has seven integrated steps for systematic monitoring and control of operations [23]:

1. Conduct a hazard analysis. Prepare a list of steps in the operational system at which significant problems or hazards can occur and identify preventive measures.
2. Identify the critical control points in the system. A critical control point is one at which control can be applied and a hazard can be prevented, eliminated, or reduced to acceptable levels.
3. Establish critical limits associated with each critical control point that would trigger enactment of preventive or corrective measures.

4. Establish critical control point monitoring requirements. Establish procedures for using monitoring results to adjust the process and maintain control of the production system.
5. Establish corrective actions to be taken when a critical limit is exceeded.
6. Establish procedures for verifying that the HACCP system is working correctly.
7. Establish effective record-keeping procedures that document the HACCP system.

Step 1: conduct a hazard analysis

Considerations for conducting a risk or hazard analysis relative to biosecurity efforts have been described in detail previously in this report. One approach to identifying points in veterinary operations at which hazards can occur is to think of the general routes of transmission for the various agents and then think more specifically about how this happens in one's own practice. For example, a problem management point relative to biosecurity controls for veterinary hospitals is the continual introduction of animals to the environment. Depending on standard procedures, this may be more problematic for chutes or outpatient facilities that are less likely to be cleaned as often as stalls. Another management problem is the shared air space for patients in enclosed hospitals. Larger hospitals such as CSU-VTH have a high potential for frequent indirect contact between patients given the large number of patients and the large number of caregivers involved in patient management.

At CSU-VTH, gastrointestinal and respiratory pathogens are probably one of the greatest nosocomial risks because animals are commonly infected with these agents, they tend to be extremely contagious, and there are numerous vectors for indirect transmission in a busy hospital environment. Another important concern is contamination and infection of surgical wounds, particularly with multidrug-resistant bacteria. In addition, specific zoonotic agents are given special consideration because of their potential for morbidity and mortality in people (e.g., rabies virus, and *Yersinia pestis* is a particular concern in the Rocky Mountains). Agents of regulatory concern also are given special priority because of the risk to normal hospital operations (e.g., vesicular stomatitis virus). Considering different agents in these categories provides a list of several important agents. As an example, a few of the agents that have been recognized as common or important threats to the patients at CSU-VTH include *Salmonella*, rabies virus, *Cryptosporidium parvum*, bovine viral diarrhea virus, bovine leukosis virus, bovine herpesvirus, equine influenza virus, equine herpesvirus, *Streptococcus equi*, canine parvovirus, *Bordatella bronchisepticum*, feline calicivirus, feline leukemia virus, feline immunodeficiency virus, *Yersinia pestis*, several ectoparasites, and foreign animal disease agents (especially vesicular stomatitis virus and foot-and-mouth disease virus).

Step 2: identify critical control points and corrective actions

Many of the critical control points for different agents are similar because of their routes of transmission. Oral-fecal transmission is a common feature of several agents of concern, such as *Salmonella*, *Cryptosporidium*, and bovine viral diarrhea virus. Similarly, aerosol transmission is a common feature among several respiratory pathogens. These transmission features need to be considered when targeting prevention efforts. In addition, hospital environments can become contaminated easily by many different agents, facilitating indirect transmission by hospital personnel. This is particularly true for agents that can persist in the environment.

General actions for breaking transmission cycles for contagious diseases should be emphasized throughout the hospital. These actions include quarantine or segregation of animals known (or suspected) to be infected with contagious pathogens, quarantine or segregation of animals with a high risk of acquiring infections, limiting intentional and circumstantial human contact with high-risk patients, and optimizing hygiene for personnel and the environment.

The large animal hospital in CSU-VTH is segregated into six distinct areas with increasing rigor for biosecurity precautions. These areas (in increasing order of precautions) are the outpatient examination and treatment areas, equine inpatient housing area, equine colic patient housing area, bovine inpatient housing and treatment areas, equine anesthesia and surgery areas, and isolation units. A specific action taken to prevent direct and indirect contact between patients includes housing animals with contagious diseases in isolation units. Animals considered to have a high risk of acquiring infections (e.g., critically ill animals and those with failure of passive transfer) also are housed separately. Personnel movement between the biosecurity areas described is limited and sometimes prohibited. Barrier nursing precautions (e.g., gloves and water-impervious gowns) are used whenever working with high-risk patients to prevent strike-through and to minimize the potential for cross-contamination between animals. Barrier gowns are assigned for use with specific patients so that clothing most likely to be contaminated essentially stays with the patient. Clinicians managing high-risk animals sometimes limit the number of people contacting patients and assign specific students to care for a specific patient and no others. Hand washing is required before handling each patient, and alcohol-based hand-sanitizing gels are available for use at other times when hand washing is not possible. Rubber boots and disinfectant footbaths are used throughout the large animal hospital. All hospital personnel that contact patients are required to wear clean, appropriate attire at all times. Protocols have been established for appropriate cleaning and disinfection of all contact surfaces, including instruments, waterers, and feeders, and also for changing all bedding, including sand, between every patient. The importance of maintaining a clean hospital environment is continually emphasized with all hospital personnel. Stalls are cleaned and thoroughly disinfected between all animals, paying particular attention to feeders, waterers, and surfaces frequently contacted by hands. Dumpsters and cleaning tools are marked for identification, and different sets are assigned for use only within specific assigned areas of the hospital. Personnel are required to store and consume food in specific areas that are separated from animal housing and handling areas to reduce the risk of zoonotic infections.

The rigor of the procedures used at CSU-VTH may not seem reasonable or feasible for smaller practices. It is possible, however, to design other protocols for limiting high-risk contact with particular patients, establishing appropriate traffic patterns in the hospital, and maintaining high levels of personal and environmental hygiene. For example, in hospitals that do not have separate isolation facilities, an animal known or suspected of having a contagious disease might be separated by leaving an empty stall between it and other patients. A standard protocol could be established to treat and examine these contagious animals after handling other lower-risk patients. Inexpensive web-based cameras could be used to monitor the general safety of patients and thereby reduce traffic through high-risk areas. Disposable gloves and separate coveralls or inexpensive disposable plastic barrier gowns (PolyWear gowns; PolyConversions, Rantoul, IL) could be assigned for use with specific patients. These barrier precautions minimize the likelihood of contaminating clothing worn around other patients. Disinfectant footbaths could be maintained outside those stalls and at other important traffic intersections.

Biosecurity in veterinary practices is fundamentally about optimizing patient care, and personal cleanliness is undisputably an important cornerstone of infection control. Contaminated hands are perhaps the most frequent route of indirect nosocomial transmission in all species [16]. The author often illustrates the common sense of this control feature with students by asking them to look closely at their hands and to consider whether they would appreciate a physician with similar cleanliness performing an examination or an invasive procedure on them.

Environmental cleanliness and waste disposal are other features that should not be overlooked in the practical application of biosecurity. Effective cleaning and disinfection are critical for breaking transmission cycles. Several reviews are available regarding disinfection recommendations for livestock facilities [4,6–8,17]. Applying copious amounts of disinfectant to dirty surfaces is not effective for decontamination. Disinfectants are quickly inactivated in the presence of even small amounts of dirt and organic debris and can be truly relied on only when applied to clean surfaces. Some disinfectants such as phenolics are more effective in the face of organic material, but they are also more likely to cause irritation with skin contact in patients or personnel. Bleach, chlorhexidine, and quaternary ammonium–based products are less irritating, but they are easily inactivated. Bedding and feces should be removed from stalls between all patients to facilitate more thorough cleaning. Physical disruption is generally required to remove gross contamination and surface films to ensure adequate disinfection. High-pressure washing can be an efficient method for cleaning large areas, but it is also possible to disseminate surface contaminants further because they may be aerosolized in the cleaning process. Cleanable surfaces should be maintained throughout practice environments wherever possible. Concrete floors are preferable to dirt, particularly for housing animals shedding contagious pathogens, because it is impossible to completely disinfect the latter. Rubber stall mats are usually quite porous, and it is difficult to maintain effective seals at edges. This was thought to be a major factor in maintenance and dissemination of *Salmonella infantis* during the 1996 outbreak at CSU-VTH [21]. Sealing or painting exposed wood and other porous surfaces greatly improves cleanability. It is important to consider quality of products and maintenance of painted surfaces when selecting sealants, however, because chipped and peeling paint provides a niche for bacterial contamination that is difficult clean. Attention also must be paid to controlling wildlife (e.g., mice and birds) and insect vectors.

Step 3: establish critical limits associated with each critical control point

Critical limits might be considered in two groups: procedural tolerances and tolerances associated with clinical and microbiologic surveillance. Procedurally, there effectively should be zero tolerance for failure of personnel to comply with established biosecurity procedures. This factor is important to consider when designing protocols. Biosecurity procedures should be rigorous enough to achieve infection control goals for the practice, but they should not be so onerous as to interfere with performance or inhibit compliance. A common barrier to compliance with more rigorous protocols are lack of appropriate resources or facilities and lack of appropriate motivation among personnel. Effective communication is essential to achieve good compliance so that personnel know *what* is expected as well as *why* these procedures are important. Formalizing protocols in written documents assists in this effort. Preparing such a document necessitates consideration of details that might be overlooked otherwise. Written documents also provide a reference for personnel to consult when there are questions, and they facilitate consistency in the event of personnel turnover. The need for some flexibility in adherence also must be considered. Despite the comprehensive and clear-cut nature of biosecurity protocols for CSU-VTH [3], the author and colleagues are continually faced with clinical situations that require special consideration and accommodation. Who will be allowed to "bend" the rules, who will authorize these deviations, and under what circumstances? An obvious situation requiring flexibility is when patient care emergencies require unusual action. We maintain a general policy that biosecurity rules should never interfere with the animal's need for immediate attention.

At CSU-VTH, there is zero tolerance for nosocomial infections in the hospital. This policy does not mean that we believe nosocomial infections will never occur, only that we are committed to all reasonable efforts necessary for prevention. For this reason, identification of all potential nosocomial infections is important. Less rigorous tolerance limits might call for identification of outbreaks rather than of every occurrence. What specifically constitutes an adverse event worthy of concern (i.e., an individual case versus a series of cases) is a matter of debate that hinges on the balance between rigor and efficiency that is appropriate for individual practices. In both instances, however, monitoring is necessary to trigger corrective action. It also should be noted that nosocomial infections resulting in clinical disease are quite often less common than subclinical infections.

Active microbiologic surveillance is not likely to be conducted in many practice settings. Passive surveillance that relies on summarization of results from clinical specimens can be used as an alternative. Depending on the virulence of the organism involved, however, a nosocomial organism can become widely disseminated in the hospital environment before a pattern in clinical disease is identified. Unfortunately, this was the case for *Salmonella* Infantis infections during the 1996 epidemic at CSU-VTH [21]

Before that outbreak, there had been no purposeful monitoring of *Salmonella* isolates obtained from hospitalized patients. Laboratory results were forwarded promptly to individual clinicians, but there was no active surveillance in other patients and no single person was responsible for compiling or summarizing results from all submissions. When it was suspected that *Salmonella* was being recovered with an unusually high frequency, a retrospective analysis of data showed that *Salmonella* Infantis was isolated from 13 equid patients during the first 5 months of 1996, and no isolates of this serotype had been obtained from CSU-VTH during all of 1995 [21]. All of these samples were submitted from animals with suspected salmonellosis, however. Active surveillance of all hospitalized patients during 7 subsequent weeks identified a much higher rate of infection; the same organism was isolated from 34 large animal patients, all of which had negative culture results at the time of admission [21]. In addition to monitoring shedding in patients, evaluating contamination of the hospital environment was critical to breaking the cycle of transmission during this outbreak, and ongoing surveillance has proven to be important in subsequent ongoing infection control efforts.

Step 4: establish critical control point monitoring requirements

As illustrated in the preceding paragraphs, it is necessary to monitor occurrences of infection or disease adequately to know when established critical limits are being exceeded. For this type of surveillance it is necessary to track both the frequency of different types of disease or infection (numerator information) and the number of patients at risk of developing these events (denominator information). Many veterinary practices do not currently use computerized records systems, other than for billing, which makes it extremely difficult to monitor and summarize diagnoses adequately for the purposes of a surveillance system. Although this system is optimal, it may not be feasible. It is possible to set up a tally system to track important numerator information over time, however. Specific categories for tallies would coincide with priorities set during the hazard analysis. Denominator information might be tracked in the same manner, or it also might be obtainable from billing records or census sheets. In larger, more complex practices, it is important to establish specifically who will track this information and how these data will be summarized and interpreted. Monitoring efforts are not efficient in these complex practices unless thorough reporting is performed by all personnel.

Meeting more stringent biosecurity goals that accompany higher levels of risk aversion often necessitate some form of active surveillance in which clinical and microbiologic data are specifically collected for biosecurity purposes, rather than for management of individual patients. It is essential to consider the specifics of what will be sampled and how it will be cultured. For example, it is one thing to decide that the stabling environment of a hospital should be monitored for contamination. It requires an entirely different level of thought to determine specifically what areas to sample, how samples will be taken, and what they will be cultured for (e.g., *Salmonella*, *Escherichia coli*, *Staphylococcus*, *Enterococcus*, and so forth). Different culture methods are required to ensure optimal sensitivity, which therefore increases the expense and difficulty of rigorously monitoring for multiple bacterial species. The interpretation of this information also must be considered. Environmental monitoring at CSU-VTH shows that it is the rule rather than the exception to isolate enteric organisms from the hospital environment and even from hands. The author and colleagues have had long-standing discussions of what this information means and when it represents a problem. We do not believe that we will be able to sterilize the entire hospital, nor do we believe that we should try. We do consider specific identification of *Salmonella* in the environment an important event, however. In this sense, *Salmonella* is important as a specific pathogen but also as a marker of general hygiene in the hospital. There should be no residual environmental source of *Salmonella*, because we expect our cleaning and disinfection procedures to eliminate these sources. In addition, environmental samples are regularly obtained from "clean" areas such as surgical suites and cultured aerobically to identify many different bacterial species, including enteric organisms. We do not expect these cultures to be sterile, but we do expect this environment to be cleaner than the stabling facility and not heavily contaminated with fecal organisms. Biosecurity personnel occasionally show up in clinical service areas unannounced and obtain swabs of hands for culture. This activity increases hygiene awareness among all personnel, and results clearly demonstrate that fecal organisms nearly always contaminate hands of personnel in the hospital except when they have been washed recently. Another aspect to consider is whether isolates are resistant to antimicrobial drugs. We routinely characterize antimicrobial resistance in isolates collected for surveillance purposes because this provides us a relatively easy method of distinguishing between isolate phenotype and looking for distribution of bacterial clones. Environmental distribution of multidrug-resistant bacteria of the same species and resistance pattern can be an indicator of a nosocomial threat. These bacteria do not have to be typical pathogens to be important, as has been discovered on numerous occasions regarding septicemias and wound infections with "resident" nosocomial organisms such as *Pseudomonas, Klebsiella, E. coli, Acinetobacter, Enterococcus, Staphylococcus, Serratia,* and so forth [1,2,9,10,15].

Monitoring for compliance with biosecurity procedures is equally important. The general tendency in all operations is for compliance with less convenient procedures to degrade over time, particularly when personnel are not fully aware or appreciative of goals and consequences. At CSU-VTH, personnel supervisors are expected to monitor and police their respective areas for compliance with biosecurity protocols, and biosecurity personnel are responsible for monitoring overall compliance with the biosecurity program. This provides a stimulus for reminding and reinforcing protocols with personnel who may have honestly forgotten to do something (or not do something). There are consequences for failing to comply with procedures, however, because biosecurity protocols are considered official hospital policy and purposeful disregard is grounds for disciplinary action.

Step 5: establish corrective actions to be taken when a critical limit is exceeded

Unless there is a will to establish corrective action when problems are recognized, there is really no need to establish a formal biosecurity program. Although this may seem obvious, good intentions for action do not necessarily predict how an operation will actually respond when a specific situation arises. Invariably, exceeding established limits for biosecurity tolerance occurs at the worst possible time logistically. It occurs when the practice is busiest, when staffing is shortest, and budgets are smallest. The long-term goal of protecting patients, personnel, and the practice should not be overshadowed by the immediacy of short-term needs, however. Allowing a formal biosecurity program to protect one's interests effectively requires that this long-range perspective be given appropriate priority.

Planning for hypothetical scenarios can help ease the burden of crisis management when triggering events are identified. For example, if one specific goal of the biosecurity program is to minimize nosocomial *Salmonella* infections, appropriate planning can help predetermine some actions that will likely be taken whenever this infection is detected. Animals known or suspected to be infected with *Salmonella* might be segregated or moved to an isolation unit. Stalls would be identified for special cleaning to minimize environmental reservoirs and may not be released for further use until negative environmental culture results were obtained. Fecal samples could be obtained daily from all animals housed near affected patients and any others considered at risk of exposure. Special diagnostic procedures such as DNA "fingerprinting" could be used to look more precisely for similarities among pertinent isolates. Increased biosecurity precautions might be initiated, such as additional footbaths, further restrictions in personnel movement, and more extensive use of barrier precautions. Appropriateness of each specific action will need to be evaluated, but usually this type of planning is helpful.

It should be noted that the most efficient method for controlling outbreaks of nosocomial disease can sometimes include drastic management procedures such as temporarily restricting or stopping new admissions. Although these drastic measures are obviously not desirable, they may be necessary to remove the fuel from the fire to stop the occurrences of new infections because the risk to new patients may be too great. It may be tempting to limp along, making all possible management changes except for temporary closure of a facility, but in the end this may not be the most efficient method of correcting the problem. Even in the absence of identifying transmissions, CSU-VTH regularly suspends or restricts admissions in various areas of CSU-VTH to facilitate depopulation and thorough top-to-bottom cleaning. We have encountered outbreak situations in both the large animal and small animal facilities, in which it was deemed most expedient and efficient to suspend activities until the problem could be corrected [21]. This action protected patients that would have been admitted from potential injury and allowed our practice to concentrate on clean-up efforts rather than carrying out separate missions for patient care and clean-up. A certain negative stigma is associated with the occurrence of outbreaks of nosocomial disease, however, which may provoke practice managers into taking a defensive posture. Unfortunately, this perception may lead practices to continue activities when it is most efficient for control to suspend admissions. This defensive position may also influence veterinarians not to be completely open about disclosure of potential risks with clients. It is almost as if veterinarians are sometimes in denial about the known risk of nosocomial infection in every hospitalized patient. Failure to disclose to clients the increased risk to patients when they are admitted during recognized outbreaks of nosocomial infection creates considerable liability for both the veterinarian and the practice, even if the incidence of new infections is low.

We maintain an open information policy at all times regarding risks for nosocomial infections at CSU-VTH. Using an informed consent form, clients are told at the time patients are admitted that nosocomial infections are one of the known risks associated with hospitalization. They also are told that fecal samples and other biologic specimens may be obtained from their horses for the purposes of surveillance. The results of these tests are fully disclosed to clients when they become available. In situations in which nosocomial infections have been identified but were believed to be under control, our standard policy is to disclose this information to clients and give them the option to seek other veterinary care if they choose. We also have encountered situations in which the stalls in our isolation facility were occupied, and the animal being admitted would normally be managed in isolation. In these situations, we believe it is better to direct clients to seek care at other referral facilities in the area or treat animals in the field rather than take unacceptable risks by not managing patients in compliance with our Biosecurity Standard Operating Procedures [3].

Step 6: establish procedures for verifying that the hazard analysis and critical control point system is working correctly

Establishing procedures for verifying that HACCP is working correctly is important for the sustained success of a biosecurity program. Procedures should be established for routine summarization and interpretation of surveillance data. There is a biosecurity committee at CSU-VTH composed of faculty and staff representatives from all hospital sections that is responsible for reviewing biosecurity activities and recommending policy actions to the hospital director. The oversight of biosecurity personnel and this committee helps to ensure that goals of the program are being met. Biosecurity committee meetings are held quarterly in which results from microbiologic surveillance, clinical incidents affecting biosecurity, and personnel compliance with biosecurity procedures are reviewed. Corrective actions are discussed and recommended, if necessary.

Step 7: establish effective record-keeping procedures

For biosecurity purposes at CSU-VTH, we are fortunate that effective operation of a large, complex referral center requires detailed record keeping of patient information and diagnostic data. It is likely that information that is useful for tracking events related to biosecurity is already being captured and archived somewhere in the hospital (e.g., medical records, financial records, pharmacy records, diagnostic laboratory data, and so forth). This may not be the case for all veterinary hospitals, and procedures must be established that allow proper recording of events affecting biosecurity, and optimally so that data can be quickly searched, retrieved, and summarized. Incident reports pertaining to biosecurity at CSU-VTH are filed routinely to archive action on specific events. Summaries of microbiologic surveillance provided to the Biosecurity Committee are maintained and updated regularly. It is also necessary to document procedures thoroughly. At CSU-VTH, biosecurity procedures are maintained in a formal standard operating procedures manual [3]. Printed copies of this manual are made available throughout the hospital and on-line [3]. Formal recording of procedures is particularly important because of the large number of people involved in the program and the annual turnover of students and other personnel.

Experience with surveillance and biosecurity at Colorado State University Veterinary Teaching Hospital

The value of surveillance and biosecurity in veterinary hospitals can be seen by reviewing experiences at CSU-VTH regarding *Salmonella* surveillance. As part of an overall biosecurity program, CSU-VTH instituted an active surveillance program in 1997 to monitor *Salmonella* shedding in large animal patients. Fecal samples are obtained at arrival from all bovine inpatients for *Salmonella* culture, as well as from all equine colic patients at arrival and every other day after that. Using this sampling scheme for 4 years, we have found that an average of approximately 18% of bovine inpatients have positive culture results at admission, and approximately 8% of colic patients have positive culture results for *Salmonella* at least once during hospitalization (average number of fecal cultures per horse = 3.1). It should be noted that the prevalence of shedding in bovine inpatients would likely be greater if a more rigorous sampling scheme were used. These data do not include culture results passively collected from animals suspected of having salmonellosis, but data from active and passive surveillance of *Salmonella* shedding are combined for monitoring of nosocomial infections. *Salmonella* isolates are characterized further regarding serogroup, serotype, and susceptibility to antimicrobial drugs. Patient information is collated regarding hospitalization dates, stabling location in the hospital, herd of origin, and other management information such as clinician of record. On about five or six occasions during these 4 years, an apparent link between *Salmonella* isolates from different patients has been identified. Longitudinal analysis of these data clearly shows that most *Salmonella* isolates are not apparently linked to temporal or geographical patterns of shedding in other hospitalized patients, however. The major exception to this statement is shedding patterns of dairy cattle from the same herd. Most cattle hospitalized at CSU-VTH are dairy animals. Isolation of *Salmonella* from beef cattle at our facility is uncommon, whereas the likelihood of shedding in dairy cattle clusters by dairy, and shedding prevalences using the sampling strategy described previously vary among different dairies from approximately 10% to 50%. In comparison, limited information gathered from other equine inpatients (not colic patients) suggests that their prevalence of *Salmonella* shedding is approximately 3% using every-other-day sampling and even lower among small animal patients (≤1%) [16]. Understanding typical shedding rates in our patients has allowed us to identify on some operations where subclinical *Salmonella* infections were endemic. This has allowed us to take special precautions with animals from these farms when they are admitted to the hospital and to assist these operations with efforts to control infections and prevent disease.

Data from the 1996 *Salmonella* outbreak suggest that nosocomial infections occurred for several months before detection. Our experience with the current surveillance program suggests that it would not be possible for similar events to occur without being detected, illustrating the tremendous power that a well-designed surveillance program can provide to biosecurity programs. Active or passive data gathering in a surveillance program is not without cost, however. Considerable effort is needed to sustain these data-gathering efforts, not to mention the costs associated with fecal cultures and subsequent susceptibility testing of *Salmonella* isolates.

It would be foolish to engage in the surveillance effort described if there were not a willingness to act on the available information. Although this may seem obvious, it is possible that monitoring activities might be enacted when a deeper consideration would show that there is an inability or unwillingness to act when these data indicate that a problem exists. The importance of surveillance findings also varies depending on the goals and risk aversion of the veterinary practice or producer. For example, although the incidence of *Salmonella* shedding among equine patients at CSU-VTH is substantially lower than the incidence in bovine patients, we find that owners of horses are generally far more risk averse regarding the consequences of *Salmonella* shedding than are owners of cattle. This may be partially attributable to differences in the consequences of *Salmonella* infections in animals, it may be somewhat related to differences in the monetary and personal value of individual animals, but it may also be attributable to differences in acceptance and familiarity with this problem. A national study of *Salmonella* shedding in dairies suggests that an average of approximately 5% of all lactating dairy cattle sampled once were found to shed *Salmonella*, and an average of approximately 18% of dairy cattle that were to be culled within a week of sampling had positive culture results [24]. Shedding prevalence varied greatly depending on season. In comparison, less than 1% of horses sampled in a similar nationwide study had positive culture results for *Salmonella* [12]. Regardless of differences in national trends among species, our obligation to all patients and clients is the same at CSU-VTH: we must strive to provide an optimal environment for animal care. We believe this means that appropriate efforts must be taken to minimize the risk of nosocomial infection in all patients.

The success of the biosecurity program is greatly dependent on participation and compliance of all personnel working at CSU-VTH, from the maintenance and cleaning crew, to the students, staff, clinicians, and administration. As such, there must be acceptance and buy-in for achieving goals for the program. Education of all personnel regarding the importance of biosecurity measures is critical to the success of biosecurity efforts so that they will know what actions are generally used to protect patients, when standard operations should change, how they change in these situations, and who to talk to if they have problems or questions. Efforts should be made to educate all personnel about the biology of important diseases whenever possible, including information about modes of transmission, the relative contagious nature of disease, shedding, persistence of agents in the environment, effective methods of disinfection, and the zoonotic potential. This knowledge allows them to better understand the importance of the program and to act wisely when specific situations require some improvisation regarding biosecurity measures.

Although participation from all personnel is critical for the success of the biosecurity program, it has been useful to have a single person with oversight responsibilities for the entire program. The author believes that this allows consistent application of biosecurity precautions for all patients, regardless of which veterinarian is responsible for patient care. If only the clinicians are responsible for ensuring application of biosecurity precautions as is true in most other hospitals, this can place veterinarians in the difficult position of attempting to provide every possible benefit to patients while protecting the best interests of the clients, in addition to protecting the practice and hospital. As discussed previously, this can create situations in which the long-term goals of the biosecurity of the program and safety of future patients can be overshadowed by the immediacy of decisions regarding the patient standing before us today. In comparison, the Director of Biosecurity at CSU-VTH is responsible for representing the interests of the hospital, which frees the veterinarian for less conflicted representation of client and patient interests. In his own role in this capacity, the author can therefore serve as an in-house consultant for biosecurity concerns regarding management of individual patients. This can actually improve the relationship between clients and the primary care veterinarian, because responsibility or "blame" for difficult management decisions pertaining to biosecurity (i.e., placing patients in isolation units, in which daily care charges to the client are greater) can be abdicated ("I feel badly about the extra charges, but our Director of Biosecurity is responsible for preventing infections in other patients, and he has decided that this move is best for all of the patients in our hospital").

We are sometimes asked by colleagues working at other veterinary practices whether our rigorous protocols and open information policy could potentially be harming the reputation of the practice. Although some might think that these actions inappropriately advertise weakness and fallibility, the author believes that our actions demonstrate an effort to achieve a higher level of patient care. In other words, our program demonstrates that our concern for patient care and personnel safety is so great that we take extra safety precautions. Who could possibly disagree with the idea that biosecurity precautions can help to reduce the risk of nosocomial infections, which in turn provides an environment where patient care is optimized? Above all, do no harm.

Acknowledgment

The author thanks all of the personnel at the Colorado State University Veterinary Teaching Hospital who have assisted in our efforts to refine and develop the biosecurity program for the hospital.

References

[1] Boerlin P, Eugster S, Gaschen F, Straub R, Schawalder P. Transmission of opportunistic pathogens in a veterinary teaching hospital. Vet Microbiol 2001;82:347–59.

[2] Colahan PT, Peyton LC, Connelly MR, Peterson R. *Serratia* spp. infection in 21 horses. J Am Vet Med Assoc 1984;185:209–11.
[3] Colorado State University Veterinary Teaching Hospital. Biosecurity standard operating procedures. Available at: http://www.cvmbs.colostate.edu/vth/unpub/biosecurity.html. Accessed 2/28/02.
[4] Dwyer RM. Disinfecting equine facilities. Rev Sci Tech 1995;14:403–18.
[5] Ezell H, Tramontin B, Hudson R, Tengelsen L, Hahn C, Smith K, et al. Outbreaks of multidrug-resistant *Salmonella typhimurium* associated with veterinary facilities: Idaho, Minnesota, and Washington, 1999. Morbidity and Mortality Weekly Report 2001;50:701–4.
[6] Ford WB. Disinfection procedures for personnel and vehicles entering and leaving contaminated premises. Rev Sci Tech 1995;14:393–401.
[7] Fotheringham VJ. Disinfection of livestock production premises. Rev Sci Tech 1995;14:191–205.
[8] Fotheringham VJ. Disinfection of stockyards. Rev Sci Tech 1995;14:293–307.
[9] Fox JG, Beaucage CM, Folta CA, Thornton GW. Nosocomial transmission of *Serratia marcescens* in a veterinary hospital due to contamination by benzalkonium chloride. J Clin Microbiol 1981;14:157–60.
[10] Glickman LT. Veterinary nosocomial (hospital-acquired) *Klebsiella* infections. J Am Vet Med Assoc 1981;179:1389–92.
[11] Glickman L, Russell H, Maher J, McCarthy M, Witte EJ, Hays CW, et al. Exposure to a rabid cow—Pennsylvania. Morbidity and Mortality Weekly Report 1983;32:128.
[12] Hill SL, Cheney JM, Taton-Allen GF, Reif JS, Bruns C, Lappin MR. Prevalence of enteric zoonotic organisms in cats. J Am Vet Med Assoc 2000;216:687–92.
[13] House JK, Mainar-Jaime RC, Smith BP, House AM, Kamiya DY. Risk factors for nosocomial *Salmonella* infection among hospitalized horses. J Am Vet Med Assoc 1999;214:1511–6.
[14] Konkle DM, Nelson KM, Lunn DP. Nosocomial transmission of *Cryptosporidium* in a veterinary hospital. J Vet Intern Med 1997;11:340–3.
[15] Koterba A, Torchia J, Silverthorne C, Ramphal R, Merritt AM, Manucy J. Nosocomial infections and bacterial antibiotic resistance in a university equine hospital. J Am Vet Med Assoc 1986;189:185–91.
[16] Larson EL. APIC guideline for handwashing and hand antisepsis in health care settings. Am J Infect Control 1995;23:251–69.
[17] Owen JM. Disinfection of farrowing pens. Rev Sci Tech 1995;14:381–91.
[18] Radostits OM, Leslie KE, Fetrow J. Record systems and herd monitoring. In: Herd health: food animal production medicine 2nd edition. Philadelphia: W.B. Saunders; 1994. p. 49–71.
[19] Reif JS, Wimmer L, Smith JA, Dargatz DA, Cheney JM. Human cryptosporidiosis associated with an epizootic in calves. Am J Public Health 1989;79:1528–30.
[20] Schott HC, Ewart SL, Walker RD, Dwyer RM, Dietrich S, Eberhart SW, et al. An outbreak of salmonellosis among horses at a veterinary teaching hospital. J Am Vet Med Assoc 2001;218:1152–9.
[21] Tillotson K, Savage CJ, Salman MD, Gentry-Weeks CR, Rice D, Fedoka-Cray PJ, et al. Outbreak of *Salmonella* infantis infection in a large animal veterinary teaching hospital. J Am Vet Med Assoc 1997;211:1554–7.
[22] Traub-Dargatz JL, Garber LP, Fedorka-Cray PJ, Ladely S, Ferris KE. Fecal shedding of *Salmonella* spp by horses in the United States during 1998 and 1999 and detection of *Salmonella* spp in grain and concentrate sources on equine operations. J Am Vet Med Assoc 2000;217:226–30.
[23] United States Department Of Agriculture. Food safety inspection service: guidebook for the preparation of haccp plans and generic haccp models. Available at http://www.fsis.usda.gov/OPPDE/nis/outreach/models/models.htm. Accessed 2/28/02.
[24] Wells SJ, Fedorka-Cray PJ, Dargatz DA, Ferris K, Green A. Fecal shedding of *Salmonella* spp. by dairy cows on farm and at cull cow markets. J Food Prot 2001;64:3–11.

Appendix
Common disinfectants used in veterinary medicine

Class	Disinfectant	Application in veterinary medicine	Activity in organic material	Comments
Acids	Acetic acid, citric acid	Disinfectant for Foot and Mouth Disease Virus	Poor	Non-toxic and non-irritating at typical dilutions.
	Lactic acid	Carcass decontamination	Poor	Non-toxic and non-irritating at typical dilutions. Immediate bactericidal effect and delayed bacteriostatic effect results in extended shelf-life of meat and decreased risk of food-borne pathogen transmission.
Alcohols	Ethanol, methanol, isopropanol	Surface disinfectant, topical antiseptic, hand sanitizing lotions.	Very poor	High concentrations for effective use in most situations as a germicide. Commercially available hand sanitizing lotions have been shown to greatly reduce bacterial counts on skin. Also effective against many viruses. Highly flammable. Irritating to injured skin, but low toxicity.
Aldehydes	Formaldehyde	Surface disinfectant, fumigant	High	Highly irritating and toxic, both through contact and fumes. Exposure to formaldehyde vapor has associated carcinogen risk. Contact sensitization can develop rapidly. Active against nonenveloped viruses, and gluteraldehyde is an effective sporocide with sufficient contact. Non-corrosive on metals, rubber, plastics, lenses, and cements. Gluteraldehyde is most active at alkaline pH.
	Gluteraldehyde	Surface disinfection and sterilization	High	
Alkalis	Sodium hydroxide (lye, soda lye)	Environmental disinfection, surface disinfectant	High	Highly caustic. Strong concentrations can be used for prion disinfection.

	Calcium hydroxide (slaked lime)	Environmental disinfection	Moderate	Sometimes used as a whitewash that kills or inhibits growth of non-spore-forming bacteria. Used extensively in Foot and Mouth Disease outbreaks.
	Sodium carbonate	Cleansing agent	Moderate	
Biguanides	Chlorhexidine	Surface disinfectant, topical antiseptic	Very poor	Very low toxicity potential. Typical dilutions are non-irritating even when contacting mucosa. Inactivated by anionic detergents. Bacteriocidal activity on skin is more rapid than many other compounds, including iodophors. Residual effect on skin diminishes regrowth.
Chlorine releasing agents	Sodium hypochlorite (Bleach)	Surface disinfectant	Very poor	Bacteriocidal activity is reduced with increasing pH, lower temperatures, and in the presence of ammonia and nitrogen compounds which can be important when urine is present. Not affected by water hardness. Considered to have relatively low toxic potential with standard dilutions. Chlorine gas can be produced when mixed with other chemicals. Strong oxidizing (bleaching) activity that can damage fabric and is corrosive on metals, silver, and aluminum (not stainless steel). Strong solutions can deactivate prion material. Chlorine dioxide is irritating and toxic.
	Calcium hypochlorite	Surface disinfectant	Very poor	
	Chlorine dioxide	Fumigant, gas sterilization	Moderate	

(continued on next page)

Appendix (*continued*)

Class	Disinfectant	Application in veterinary medicine	Activity in organic material	Comments
Iodine releasing agents	Iodine solutions	Surface disinfectant, topical antiseptic	Very poor	Absorption of iodine and associated toxicity is greatest with tinctures and solutions, and reduced with iodophores. People can become sensitized to skin contact. Generally less active than chlorine releasing agents. Bacteriocidal activity is slowed at lower temperatures and alkaline pH, but affected less by organic material than chlorine releasing agents.
	Iodophors	Surface disinfectant, topical antiseptic	Very poor	Dilution of iodophors increases free iodine concentration and antimicrobial activity. Metal surfaces can be oxidized. Staining of tissues and plastics also occurs.
Peroxygens	Peroxymonosulfate	Surface disinfectant, fumigant	High	Low toxic potential and non-irritating. No harmful decomposition products.
	Hydrogen peroxide	Surface disinfectant, topical antiseptic, gas sterilization	Low	Peroxymonosulfate is labeled for use against Foot and Mouth Disease Virus, and can be used in the presence of animals. Peracetic acid (PAA) may be a weak carcinogen. Hydrogen peroxide (HP) has brief germicidal activity when applied to tissues. Poor lipid solubility. Less active at low temperatures. Excellent against spores.
	Peracetic acid	Surface disinfectant fumigant	High	PAA is germicidal at much lower concentrations than HP. Corrosive to plain steel, iron, copper, brass, bronze, and vinyl, and rubber.

Phenols	Various phenols (2-phenylphenol, benzylphenol, 4-chloro-3,5-dimethylphenol, etc.)	Surface disinfectant	High	Irritation is variable among compounds, but these compounds are in general highly irritating and should not be used on surfaces that contact skin or mucosa. Environmental safety is also variable. Not affected by hardness of water. Extended residual activity after drying. Active against non-enveloped viruses. Some residual activity after drying.
Quaternary ammonium compounds	Various ammonium salts (mono-alkyltrimethyl ammonium salts, etc.)	Surface disinfectant	Moderate	Irritation and toxicity is variable among products, but these compounds are generally non-irritating and have low toxicity at typical dilutions. Inactivated by anionic detergents. Some residual activity after drying. Good hard water tolerance, more effective at alkaline pH.

Data from Block SS, editor. Disinfection, sterilization, and preservation, 5th edition. Philidelphia: Lippincott Williams and Wilkins; 2001; and Linton AH, Hugo WB, Russell AD, editors. Disinfection in veterinary and farm animal practice. Oxford: Blackwell Scientific Publications; 1987.

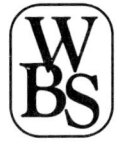

Vet Clin Food Anim 18 (2002) 157–175

THE VETERINARY
CLINICS
Food Animal
Practice

Epidemiologic tools for biosecurity and biocontainment

David R. Smith, DVM, PhD

*Department of Veterinary and Biomedical Sciences,
Institute of Agriculture and Natural Resources,
University of Nebraska–Lincoln, Lincoln, NE 68583–0907, USA*

The goal of a biosecurity or biocontainment plan is to prevent the transmission of infectious agents among individuals, groups of animals, farms, or geopolitical regions [10,16,19]. The principles of biosecurity and biocontainment are to increase the resistance of the host, eliminate reservoirs of the agent, and prevent contacts that result in transmission. The host, agent, and environmental circumstances under which these principles could be applied might vary considerably, so the specific strategies used to apply these principles also might vary in usefulness or efficiency depending on the circumstances.

In some cases, biosecurity or biocontainment strategies that seem like a good idea are ineffective or inefficient in practice. Fundamental epidemiologic principles and the probability theory have been used to model the expected outcomes of biosecurity or biocontainment actions before the actions are implemented.

Quantitative models

Models are carefully selected abstractions of reality. Quantitative models represent concepts mathematically [6]. Biosecurity or biocontainment strategies can be evaluated by modeling quantitative epidemiologic relationships (formulas describing how infectious disease parameters interact in populations) using computer software programs. The uses for quantitative modeling are endless; the examples in this article illustrate how models can be useful for evaluating varying biosecurity scenarios or conceptualizing how the various parameters of a biosecurity strategy might interact.

Corresponding author. 124 Veterinary Diagnostic Center, PO Box 830907, Lincoln, NE 68583–0907, USA.

E-mail address: dsmith8@unl.edu (D.R. Smith).

To use the concepts presented in this article, the reader must become familiar with common computer spreadsheet functions, including how to enter formulas and how to create graphs. Computer spreadsheet software programs are now sufficiently user-friendly so that quantitative analysis is within the grasp of anyone with interest. It is also necessary to become familiar with the quantitative epidemiologic relationships appropriate to the situation, many of which have been described in textbooks and journal articles. The examples in this article were prepared using readily available commercial spreadsheet software (Excel 97, Microsoft Corp., Redmond, WA; Quattro Pro9, Corel Corp., Ottawa, Ontario, Canada).

Veterinarians can use quantitative models to "test-drive" biosecurity plans within a variety of "what-if" scenarios. Models are not a substitute for clinical judgment; rather, the modeling process complements clinical judgment to enhance the decision-making process. The analysis and interpretation of a quantitative model are only as good as the clinical judgment brought to bear on the information [17].

Models range in complexity, but often even simple models are useful. Of course, a quantitative model is only as reliable as the assumptions and data used to prepare it. Models never fully represent reality; however, they can be useful tools to help one think through the process and evaluate how various parameters may influence the outcome of the actions planned [17]. Because quantitative models are concise numeric expressions of probability, the confusion of less useful subjective expressions (e.g., "that could happen") are avoided [2].

The inputs of a quantitative model are variables that can be controlled and parameters that are inherent and uncontrollable. For example, a model of a diagnostic test strategy may have inputs of sample size, which is controllable, and parameters for test performance (e.g., sensitivity and specificity), which may not be controllable. The output of a model may be measures of goal attainment or other useful outcomes [6].

Quantitative models may be deterministic or stochastic. Deterministic models assume that all of the parameters of the model are known. In stochastic models, some elements of the model are not known with certainty [6]. The examples presented in this article represent deterministic modeling. In some situations it is difficult to build a reasonable deterministic model because of the uncertainty of some parameters. In these cases, stochastic (simulation) models may be more appropriate [20]. Simulation models can be powerful tools for prediction; however, even simulation requires knowledge of the distributions of the underlying parameters, which are seldom known with accuracy [2].

A model is valid when it behaves as the object it represents in every relevant way [3]. Efforts should be made to demonstrate that predictions from quantitative models fit real observations. This advice has obvious limitations; if the observational data for validation were always available, there would be no need for the model [3].

Modeling diagnostic tests

Diagnostic tests are used to promote biosecurity and biocontainment by identifying reservoirs of disease or infection within a herd, preventing the introduction of infected animals into a herd, and assessing the level of existing infection within a herd. Throughout this article, the terms *infection* and *disease* are used as if they were synonymous to avoid unnecessary confusion. Of course, infection is not synonymous with disease, and the reader is cautioned to understand the distinction.

Diagnostic tests are not perfect, and some test results can be expected to be in error. Diagnostic test evaluation predicts what errors might occur among diseased and nondiseased populations, and diagnostic test interpretation predicts how the errors might be distributed among populations that test positive or negative. This information can be used to predict the effect that diagnostic errors might have on a test-based biosecurity plan.

Diagnostic test evaluation

Diagnostic test performance is evaluated by the parameters of sensitivity and specificity [11,12]. Sensitivity and specificity are estimated by testing individuals of known (or suspected) disease (or infection) status. Sensitivity (*SENS*) is a conditional probability describing the probability that a diseased individual (*D*+) will have a positive test result (*T*+). It is important to note that the probability is expressed for the population of individuals with disease.

$$SENS = P(T+ \,|D+)$$

Specificity (*SPEC*) is the conditional probability that a nondiseased (D−) individual will test negative (T−). The probability only applies to the population of individuals without disease.

$$SPEC = P(T- \,|D-)$$

Diagnostic test interpretation

Sensitivity and specificity values by themselves are not useful for test interpretation because practitioners do not know the true disease status of the animals they test. Practitioners are most interested in the probability that the test result represents the true infection status of the individual. This probability is called the *post-test probability* or *predictive value* [11,12]. Positive predictive value (*PPV*) is the conditional probability that an individual with a positive test result is truly infected. Negative predictive value (*NPV*) is the conditional probability that an individual with a negative test result is not truly infected.

$$PPV = P(D+ \,|T+)$$
$$NPV = P(D- \,|T-)$$

Experienced practitioners know intuitively that clinical judgment is necessary to interpret diagnostic test results. The importance of clinical judgment to test interpretation can be shown in quantitative models. Post-test probability is calculated by using information about test sensitivity and specificity as well as information called *pre-test probability*. Pre-test probability is the probability of the individual truly being diseased (P_D) before considering test results. One could think of P_D as the proportion of animals that actually has a specific disease from an imaginary population of animals, all with the same clinical presentation and history. Practitioners estimate P_D using what is known from review of the literature (e.g., from surveys reporting prevalence), history and physical examination, or previous experience. The formulas for PPV and NPV in terms of SENS, SPEC, and P_D are as follows [12]:

$$PPV = \frac{SENS \times P_D}{(SENS \times P_D) + (1 - SPEC) \times (1 - P_D)}$$

$$NPV = \frac{SPEC \times (1 - P_D)}{SPEC \times (1 - P_D) + (1 - SENS) \times P_D}$$

Creating a spreadsheet model

These formulas can be used to model the effect of test performance and clinical judgment (i.e., pre-test probability) on test interpretation (i.e., post-test probability). An ELISA test to detect antibodies directed against *Mycobacterium paratuberculosis* has been reported to have a range of SENS values (15.4%–88.1%), depending on the clinical presentation, and a SPEC of approximately 96.8% [5]. It can be assumed, based on this information, that the ELISA is 80% sensitive for infected adult cattle exhibiting clinical signs, and 25% sensitive for infected adult cattle with no clinical signs and that the test is 97% specific.

The spreadsheet model is created by first entering the values for SENS and SPEC into separate cells at the top of the spreadsheet (first for adult cattle with clinical signs, later for adult cattle without clinical sings) and, in a row of cells, entering a series of values ranging from 0 to 1 to represent a range of values for P_D. Below each of the values for P_D, the formula for PPV is entered, and below that the formula for NPV. The values visible in the formula cells represent the solution to the formula (Fig. 1A). The values for PPV and NPV are graphed (y axis) against the values for P_D (x axis) (Fig. 1B).

Examples

Predictive value

After considering the history of and physical examination findings for the animal, and based on his or her own previous experience with the disease, a veterinary practitioner determines that the probability of Johne's disease is

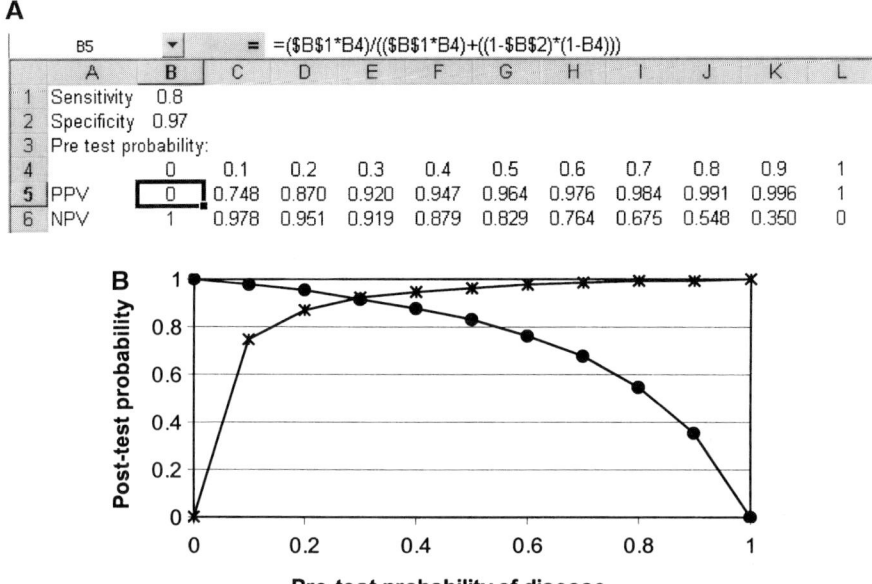

Fig. 1. Spreadsheet (A) and graphic (B) models of negative (NPV, circle) and positive (PPV, ex) predictive value for test results from adult cattle exhibiting clinical signs of Johne's disease, with different estimates of pretest probability of disease (P_D) based on a test sensitivity of 80% and test specificity of 97%.

40% for the adult cow just examined with chronic diarrhea (e.g., the veterinarian supposes that 40% of the imaginary population of animals exactly like this cow would have Johne's disease). A blood sample is collected for ELISA. The model (Fig. 1B) shows that if the test result is positive, the probability that the animal truly has the disease is 95%; the test has helped the veterinarian become more confident in a diagnosis of Johne's disease. If the test result were negative, the probability that the animal is truly not infected is 88% (i.e., the same as a 12% probability of infection); this number is below the veterinarian's estimate of the pre-test probability of disease and emphasizes that other differential diagnoses also should be considered.

The model of predictive value helps one to understand the importance of applying clinical judgment as test results are interpreted. Note that as P_D increases from 0 to 1, PPV increases from 0 to 1, and NPV decreases from 1 to 0. The model shows that test results can either be completely reliable or completely erroneous, and for a given test, the ability to estimate pretest probability accurately (i.e., apply clinical judgment) is the factor that allows reasonable interpretation of test results. With the practitioner's increased confidence that the animal is infected, the probability that a positive test result reflects the true infection status of the animal increases, and the probability that a negative test result reflects the true infection status decreases.

How does test performance affect the model? If the performance values for tests of adult cattle without clinical signs (25% SENS and 97% SPEC) are entered into the spreadsheet, the shape of the curves for PPV and NPV changes in the graphic model (Fig. 2). In particular, the curve representing NPV flattens out so that NPV is similar to the value of $(1 - P_D)$. In other words, the probability of a test-negative animal being infected $(1 - NPV)$ is near what was predicted before testing (P_D). If the model is correct, it is expected that negative ELISA results of nonclinical adult cattle provide little new information about the infection status of the animal.

Prepurchase testing

If, as the model shows, a negative ELISA test result is not informative, then this may have implications for a Johne's disease biosecurity program based on testing individuals. According to a national survey [15], dairy farmers purchasing healthy adult cattle at random from the population of US dairy cattle might expect 3.4% of the purchased cattle to be infected with *M. paratuberculosis*. If the cattle were purchased only after confirming that their ELISA test results were negative, then, from the model, one would expect 2.7% of the purchased cattle to be infected. After studying the model, the farmer and veterinarian could decide if prepurchase testing of cattle was a cost-effective biosecurity measure against introducing Johne's disease to the herd through purchased adult cattle.

Modeling the results from surveys

Apparent prevalence

Quantitative models can be used to predict the outcomes of surveys for disease prevalence. Apparent prevalence *(AP)* is the percentage of animals determined to be diseased (infected) based on diagnostic test results [11]. Apparent prevalence may differ from true prevalence because of test error.

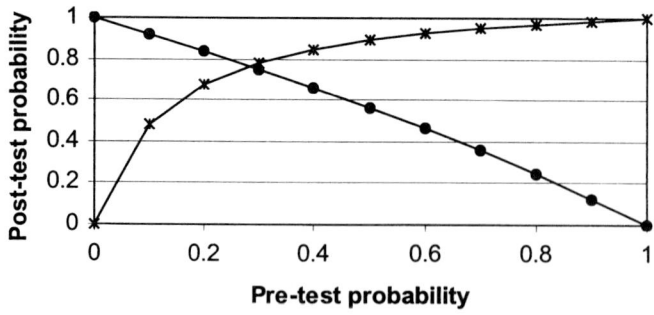

Fig. 2. Graphic model of NPV and PPV for test results from adult cattle not exhibiting clinical signs of Johne's disease, with different estimates of P_D based on a test sensitivity of 25% and test specificity of 97%.

If the parameters of test performance are known, then AP can be predicted over a range of values for true prevalence (P_D):

$$AP = SENS \times P_D + (1 - SPEC) \times (1 - P_D)$$

Diagnostic efficiency

Tests may have false-positive or false-negative results. False-negative (*FN*) results are a function of SENS (FN = 1 − SENS), and false-positive (*FP*) results are a function of SPEC (FP = 1 − SPEC). Diagnostic efficiency (*EFFIC*) describes the percentage of individuals correctly classified by the test results. Diagnostic efficiency depends on the parameters of test performance and P_D [18].

$$EFFIC = SENS \times P_D + SPEC \times (1 - P_D)$$

Example

Prevalence surveys

Based on the model of AP, if a practitioner planned to survey a random sample of nonclinical adult cattle for antibodies against *M. paratuberculosis* using ELISA serology, he or she would expect to overestimate the prevalence of disease (i.e., AP:P_D ratio >1) in populations in which the infection is rare and underestimate the prevalence in populations in which it is common (Fig. 3A and B). From the model of EFFIC, a greater percentage of individuals would be classified correctly in surveys of low-prevalence populations compared with surveys of higher-prevalence populations (Fig. 3A and C). Investigators might find these models useful for planning prevalence surveys.

Modeling the probability of an event

Animals originating from other herds present an important biosecurity risk for many infectious livestock diseases [16,19]. Biosecurity programs should therefore consider the probability that herd additions will introduce dangerous or economically damaging infectious agents.

Examples

Bovine viral diarrhea virus biosecurity

A dairy heifer grower is concerned about purchasing animals that are persistently infected with bovine viral diarrhea virus (BVDV-PI), because even one BVDV-PI animal increases the risk to the group for respiratory disease morbidity, reproductive failure, and the generation of additional BVDV-PI fetuses [10,14]. In this case, the heifer grower is able to rear as many as 300 heifers in a segregated group. Assuming that the probability of purchasing a BVDV-PI dairy heifer (P_D) is 0.01 (Bruce Brodersen, DVM,

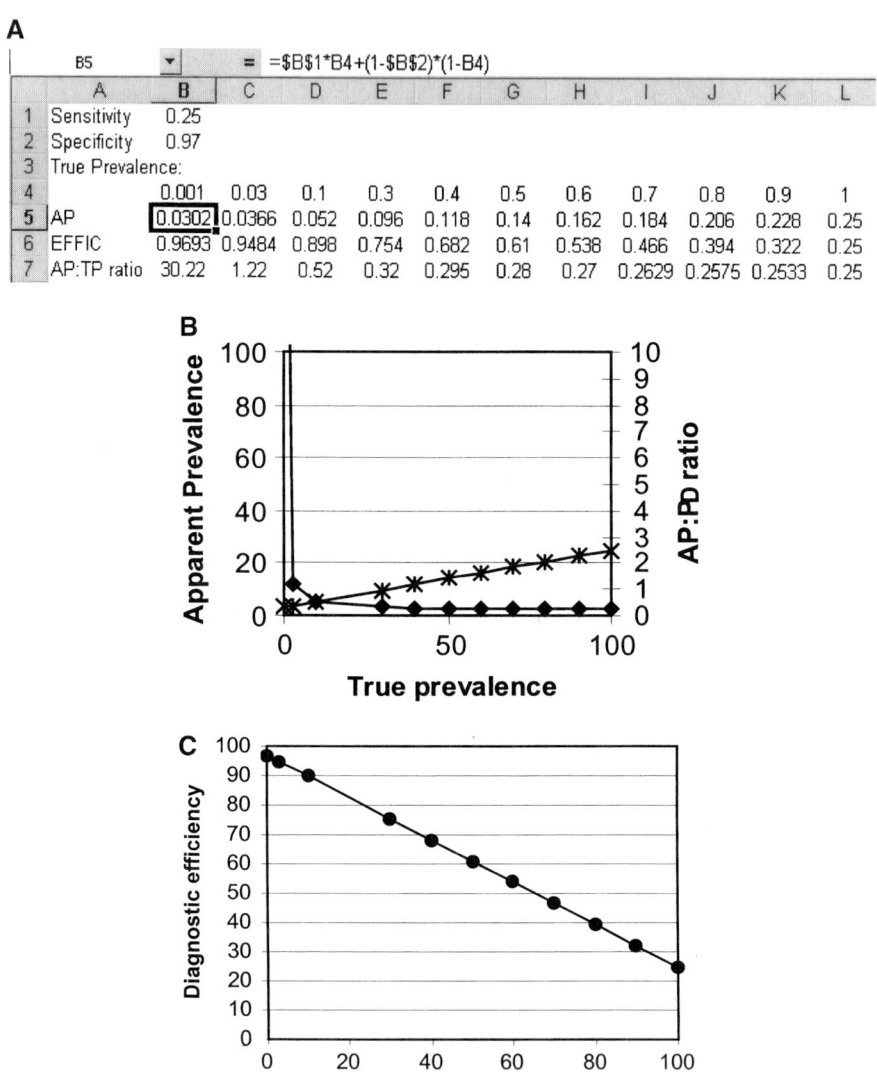

Fig. 3. Spreadsheet (A) and graphic (B) models of the apparent prevalence (AP) and the diagnostic efficiency (EFFIC, C) for different values of true prevalence (P_D) based on a test sensitivity of 25% and test specificity of 97%. Ex = AP, diamond = AP:P_D ratio.

PhD, Lincoln, NE, personal communication, May 2001), what biosecurity practices could be implemented in this operation to reduce the total number of heifers exposed to BVDV-PI carriers?

How likely is the presence of one or more BVDV-PI heifers in a group of 300? If the heifer grower purchases randomly from the general population of dairy heifers, then the number of BVDV-PI heifers present in any given group might be predicted to occur following the pattern of a binomial probability distribution [4,21]. Binomial probabilities are defined by the number of trials (e.g., 300 heifers) and the probability of an event for each trial (e.g., each heifer has 0.01 probability of being BVDV-PI).

Most computer spreadsheets have functions to calculate binomial probability distributions. The probability of the event ($P_D = 0.01$) and the number of trials (300) are entered into separate cells, and integers 0 to 10 are entered into a row of cells to represent the range of BVDV-PI animals that might be found within the group. The functions for the binomial distribution are entered in the row below the integers (Fig. 4A).

The most common number of BVDV-PI animals expected in a group of 300 is 3 (3 BVDV-PI animals expected to occur in 22.5% of the groups, Fig. 4B). It would be extremely rare to observe 10 BVDV-PI animals in a group of 300 (i.e., expected in 0.1% of groups), and 5% of the heifer groups would be expected to have no BVDV-PI. Conversely, 95% of the groups are expected to include one or more BVDV-PI animals, so 95% of the heifers raised in this production system would be expected to have exposure to BVDV-PI animals.

Because it is expected that a single BVDV-PI animal presents sufficient exposure to the entire group to cause undesirable health outcomes, the practitioner is interested in a biosecurity strategy that would result in the greatest

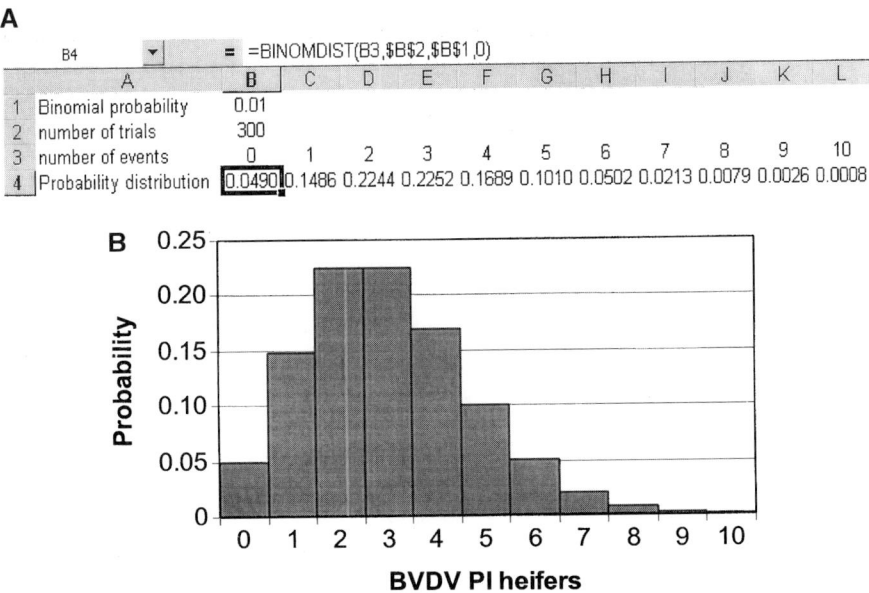

Fig. 4. Spreadsheet (A) and graphic (B) models of the binomial probability of acquiring various numbers of animals persistently infected with bovine viral diarrhea virus (BVDV-PI) in a group of 300, if the probability of BVDV-PI in the population was 0.01.

percentage of groups without BVDV-PI animals. The inputs of the binomial model make it clear that the percentage of groups without BVDV exposure is a function of (1) the number of heifers (i.e., trials) per group, and (2) the probability that a heifer is a BVDV-PI animal (i.e., the probability of the event for each trial).

Controlling group size

First, one models the percentage of groups predicted to be without BVDV-PI animals with a variety of smaller group sizes. The model is created in the spreadsheet by defining the P_D of a BVDV-PI animal as 0.01, varying the number of animals congregated into a pen from 1 to 300 (representing the number of binomial trials), and using a formula to determine the probability of one or more BVDV-PI animals within the group $[(P(x \geq 1|n, p) = 1 - P(x = 0|n, p)]$. If the number of animals congregated within a pen is reduced, the probability of the pen containing a BVDV-PI animal decreases (Fig. 5A and B). One could use this information to choose a pen size to achieve an acceptable proportion of pens exposed to BVDV-PI cattle.

Prepurchase testing

Another strategy to reduce the probability that the group includes a BVDV-PI heifer is to test the heifers before purchase and allow only test-negative animals onto the premises. Microscopic examination of skin biopsies stained by immunohistochemistry to detect BVDV-PI animals is

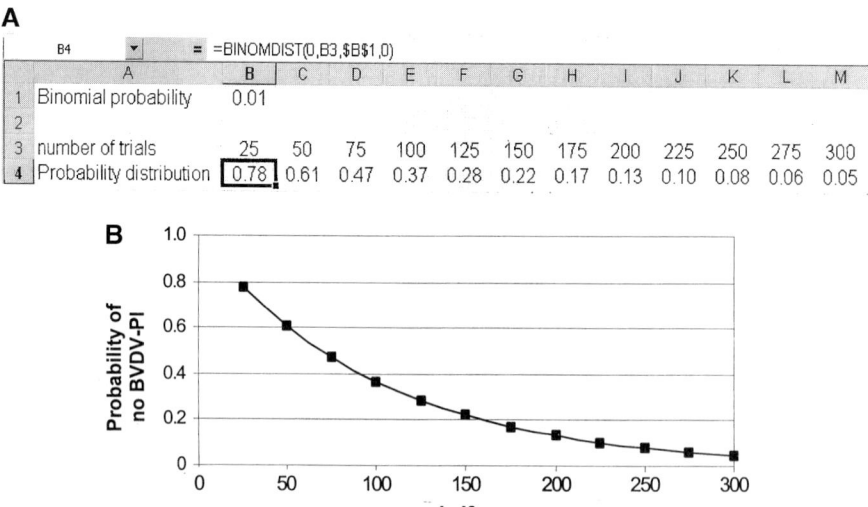

Fig. 5. Spreadsheet (A) and graphic (B) models of the binomial probability that groups of varying sizes would contain no BVDV-PI animals, if the cattle were acquired from a population with a probability of BVDV-PI equal to 0.01.

reported to be 99% sensitive and 99.9% specific (Bruce Brodersen, DVM, PhD, Lincoln, NE, personal communication, May 2001). Given these values for test performance and P_D of 0.01, one would expect 99.99% of test-negative heifers to be truly negative (NPV = 0.9999). Conversely, the probability of a test-negative BVDV-PI heifer would be 0.0001. The binomial model shows that the probability of having no BVDV-PI animals in a pen of 300 is 0.97 if the individual probability of a BVDV-PI from test-negative animals is 0.0001 (Fig. 6). If the assumptions of the model are correct, then prepurchase screening tests might prevent BVDV-PI exposure to 97% of the pens of 300 cattle, and therefore prepurchase screening for BVDV-PI as a biosecurity strategy could be extremely effective.

Considering subpopulations

Prepurchase testing might not always be the best way to reduce P_D. The value of P_D could vary widely from source to source depending on the exposure and biosecurity practices of each herd of origin, so, strategies to avoid purchasing infected animals also should consider the history of the specific subpopulation. With accurate assumptions regarding P_D based on knowledge of the subpopulation of origin, the probability of purchasing infected animals from herds with different values for P_D could be modeled over a range of numbers of animals purchased. Consider Johne's disease again as an example.

A dairy considering expansion could purchase adult cattle from several subpopulations that might vary in the P_D expected for cattle with *M. paratuberculosis* infection. The dairy might purchase (1) cattle from herds free of Johne's disease ($P_D = 0$); (2) cattle from herds with Johne's disease (assume $P_D = 0.15$); (3) cattle randomly selected from the general population of herds with and without Johne's disease (assume 22% of dairies are infected × P_D of

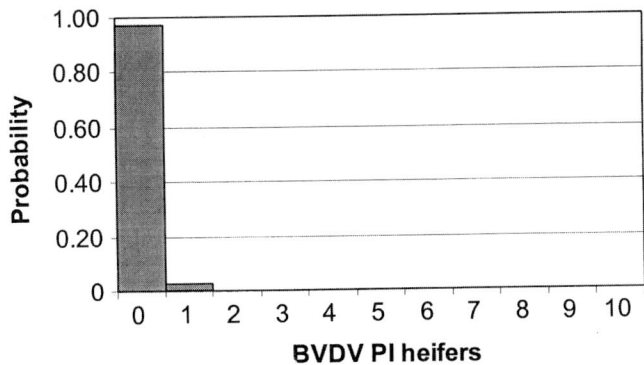

Fig. 6. Graphic model of the binomial probability of acquiring various numbers of BVDV-PI animals in a group of 300 test-negative cattle, if the probability of BVDV-PI in the population of test-negative cattle (NPV) was 0.0001.

0.15 within infected herds = overall P_D = 0.034) [15]; (4) ELISA-negative cattle from the general population (P_D = 1 – NPV = 0.027); (5) cattle from herds achieving level 2 of the US Voluntary Johne's Disease Herd Status Program for Cattle [1] (JDHSP) (5% of level 2 herds diseased × P_D of 0.05 within infected herds = overall P_D = 0.0025); or (6) cattle from herds achieving JDHSP level 3 (2% of level 2 herds diseased × P_D of 0.05 within infected herds = overall P_D = 0.001).

If the dairy could purchase cattle only from Johne's disease–free herds (an unrealistic assumption), there would be no risk of purchasing *M. paratuberculosis*–infected animals regardless of the number of animals purchased (P_D = 0). For the remaining subpopulations, there is some probability of infection (P_D > 0), and so the binomial probability of purchasing an infected animal as the number of purchased cattle increases can be modeled.

One can compare the risk associated with purchasing cattle from the various subpopulations by modeling the probability that at least one infected animal would be included with varying numbers of cattle purchased from the various subpopulations. The probability of purchasing infected cattle from the level 2 and 3 herds of cattle is much less than that of purchasing from the other subpopulations (Fig. 7). Note that the probability of purchasing an infected animal after prepurchase testing was only marginally less than if purchasing from the general population. This relationship is explained by the previous model (see Fig. 2) showing that the post-test probability of *M. paratuberculosis* infection (1 – NPV) was nearly equal to the pre-test probability of infection (P_D) when testing clinically normal adult cattle. In this case, the model helps one to visualize that knowing the individual's test status was not as useful as knowing the status of the herd of origin.

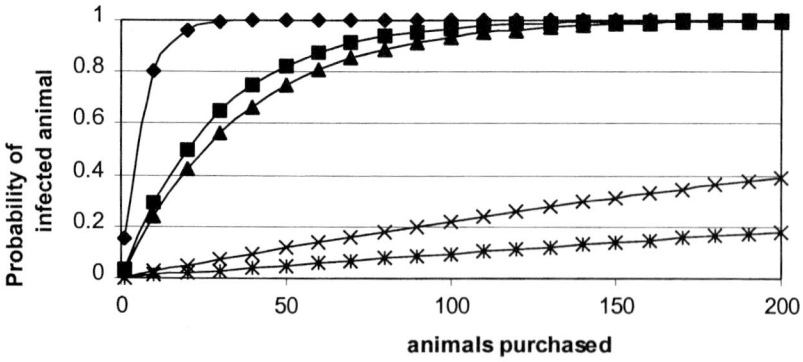

Fig. 7. Graphic model of the binomial probability that at least one *M. paratuberculosis*–infected animal would be among varying numbers of cattle purchased from subpopulations with different probabilities of infection. Diamond = infected herd; square = general population; triangle = test negative from general population; ex = level 2 herd; double ex = level 3 herd.

Modeling aggregate testing strategies

Sometimes it is important to determine if a disease is present or absent within an aggregate of individuals, for example, a litter, pen, barn, flock, or herd (the term *herd* is used to designate any such group of animals). The US Voluntary JDHSP [1] is an example of a strategy to define the infection status of the herd based on testing individuals. The probability of detecting evidence of disease or infection in a diseased herd is termed *herd-level sensitivity* (*HSENS*). If the disease status of a herd is determined by testing individuals, then HSENS is a function of SENS, SPEC, P_D, the number of reactors used to classify the herd as infected, the size of the herd, and the number of animals tested within the herd [8,13]. If there is an expected minimum value for P_D within infected herds and test performance has been evaluated, then the number of animals to test can be determined to ensure a given value for HSENS. This value is the number of animals that must be tested to detect the presence of infection with a probability equal to HSENS [13].

Herds could be classified based on different cut-point values for the numbers of reactors (*R*) used to classify the herd as diseased. HSENS can be estimated using the binomial probability distribution given the probability of a given number of reactors being present in a sample of size n from the herd. The probability of a reactor is the sum of the probability of a true positive reactor (SENS $\times P_D$) plus the probability of a false-positive reactor $[(1 - \text{SPEC}) \times (1 - P_D)]$; this is the AP, as previously defined.

Except for the unusual circumstance when a test of individuals is perfectly specific (SPEC = 1), it is possible for false-positive reactors (FP = 1 – SPEC) to result in a false-positive herd classification. It is evident that consideration also must be given to herd-level specificity (*HSPEC*), the probability that the nondiseased herd would be classified correctly [13].

Often the sample size (n) is large relative to the herd size (N) (n/N > 0.05), and usually herd sampling is conducted without replacement (i.e., once tested, the animal is removed from the pool for selection). In these circumstances, the hypergeometric distribution function is more appropriate for calculating HSENS and HSPEC [8]. Calculation of the hypergeometric function requires inputs for R, n, N, and the number of infected animals in the herd (S).

$$\text{HSENS} = 1 - P(x < R | n, p = \text{AP in a diseased herd})$$

(Binomial distribution)

$$= 1 - P[x < R | n, S = (N \times \text{AP}), N] \text{(Hypergeometric distribution)}$$

$$\text{HSPEC} = P[x < R | \text{sample size} = n, p = (1 - \text{SPEC})]$$

(Binomial distribution)

$$= P[x < R | n, S = N \times (1 - \text{SPEC}), N]$$

(Hypergeometric distribution)

Models for herd-level positive and negative predictive value (HPV+, HPV−), apparent prevalence (HAP), and diagnostic efficiency (HEFFIC) can be developed by substituting HSENS for SENS, HSPEC for SPEC, and the proportion of herds with infected individuals (HP$_D$) for P$_D$ into the appropriate formulas [13]. Simulation models for herd-level test performance have also been described [9].

Example

Herd surveillance

The assumption is made, as before, that ELISA serology used to identify nonclinical *M. paratuberculosis*–infected cattle is 25% sensitive, 97% specific, and that 22% of herds are diseased. Also assume that if a herd is diseased, then at least 5% of the adult cattle within the herd are infected.

A sample size of at least 60 cattle from a diseased herd of 200 must be tested to have a 95% probability of detecting at least one ELISA-positive reactor (HSENS = 0.95, Fig. 8A and B). Unfortunately, if that many cattle from a nondiseased herd were tested, it would be likely that false-positive ELISA results would result in false-positive herd classifications (HSPEC = 0.11, Fig. 8A and B). Only 23% of the herds classified as diseased truly would be diseased (Fig. 8C). If this strategy was used to survey the population, it would seem that 90% of herds were diseased, and only 30% of the herds would have been classified correctly (Fig. 8D). Although SENS of the ELISA is low, the model helps one to see that SPEC must be improved to make the herd-testing strategy useful.

The herd test parameters would change dramatically (Fig. 9A) if the testing strategy were changed so that the feces from cattle with ELISA-positive results were tested next by culture, resulting in an overall test performance of SENS = 0.15 and SPEC = 0.9999. In this serial testing strategy, SENS was sacrificed to improve SPEC [12]. With sufficient sample size, however, the model predicts that it would be possible to achieve >95% values for HPV+, HPV−, and HEFFIC, and HAP approaches the true herd prevalence (Fig. 9B and C). Subpopulations of herds with different risk factors for Johne's disease might have different expected values for P$_D$ and HP$_D$ [7]. The model can be configured to show that most herds for which this herd-testing strategy was used would be classified correctly (HEFFIC >90%) over a wide range of values for P$_D$ and HP$_D$, and it also would point out the conditions when the test strategy would be less efficient (low P$_D$ and high HP$_D$, Fig. 10).

The choice of sample size does have important implications for herd surveillance and survey research. Careful study of this model would show that the outcome of surveys to detect diseased herds may be biased if sample size estimates failed to consider the effect of imperfect test performance, herd size, and clustering of disease in subpopulations [13]. Sample size estimates are often obtained from software that uses formulas assuming perfect test performance; however, the model shows that serious errors in sample size estimation can result if test performance is not considered. The model also illustrates that for a given sample size, the accuracy of the herd's disease

A

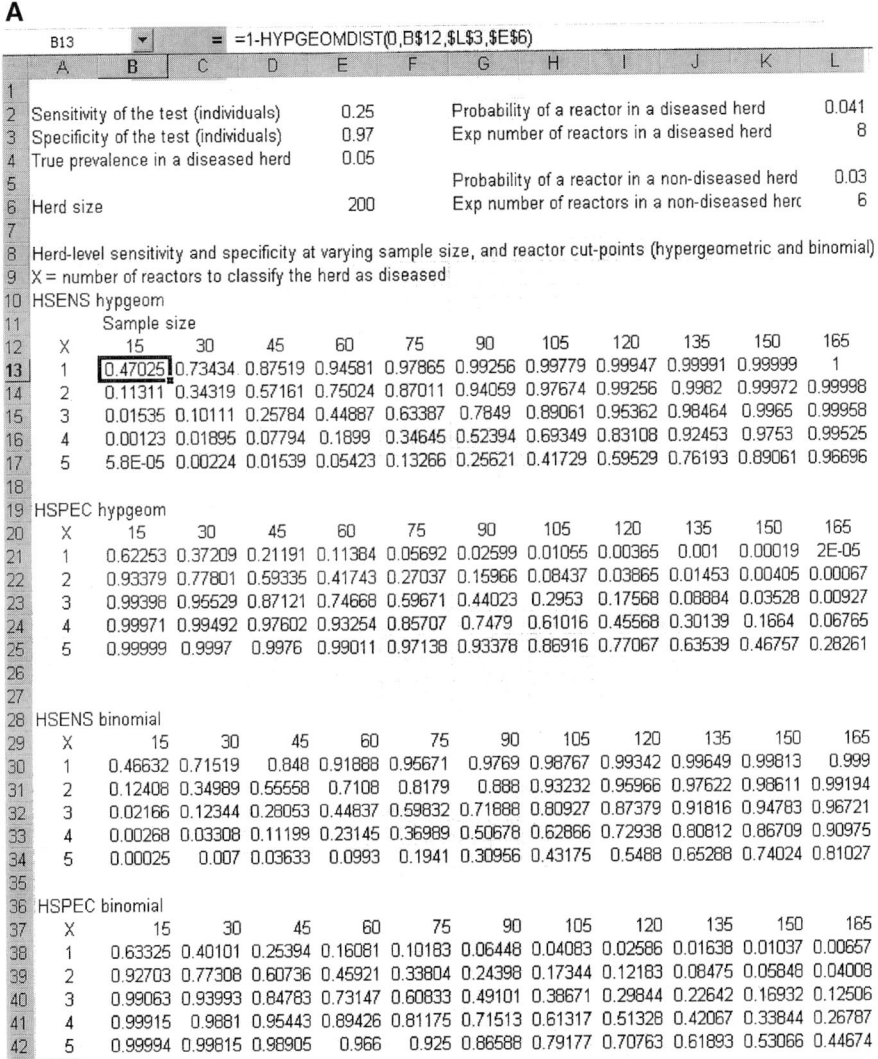

| B13 | ▼ | = | =1-HYPGEOMDIST(0,B$12,$L$3,$E$6) |

	A	B	C	D	E	F	G	H	I	J	K	L
1												
2	Sensitivity of the test (individuals)				0.25		Probability of a reactor in a diseased herd					0.041
3	Specificity of the test (individuals)				0.97		Exp number of reactors in a diseased herd					8
4	True prevalence in a diseased herd				0.05							
5							Probability of a reactor in a non-diseased herd					0.03
6	Herd size				200		Exp number of reactors in a non-diseased herd					6
7												
8	Herd-level sensitivity and specificity at varying sample size, and reactor cut-points (hypergeometric and binomial)											
9	X = number of reactors to classify the herd as diseased											
10	HSENS hypgeom											
11		Sample size										
12	X	15	30	45	60	75	90	105	120	135	150	165
13	1	0.47025	0.73434	0.87519	0.94581	0.97865	0.99256	0.99779	0.99947	0.99991	0.99999	1
14	2	0.11311	0.34319	0.57161	0.75024	0.87011	0.94059	0.97674	0.99256	0.9982	0.99972	0.99998
15	3	0.01535	0.10111	0.25784	0.44887	0.63387	0.7849	0.89061	0.95362	0.98464	0.9965	0.99958
16	4	0.00123	0.01895	0.07794	0.1899	0.34645	0.52394	0.69349	0.83108	0.92453	0.9753	0.99525
17	5	5.8E-05	0.00224	0.01539	0.05423	0.13266	0.25621	0.41729	0.59529	0.76193	0.89061	0.96696
18												
19	HSPEC hypgeom											
20	X	15	30	45	60	75	90	105	120	135	150	165
21	1	0.62253	0.37209	0.21191	0.11384	0.05692	0.02599	0.01055	0.00365	0.001	0.00019	2E-05
22	2	0.93379	0.77801	0.59335	0.41743	0.27037	0.15966	0.08437	0.03865	0.01453	0.00405	0.00067
23	3	0.99398	0.95529	0.87121	0.74668	0.59671	0.44023	0.2953	0.17568	0.08884	0.03528	0.00927
24	4	0.99971	0.99492	0.97602	0.93254	0.85707	0.7479	0.61016	0.45568	0.30139	0.1664	0.06765
25	5	0.99999	0.9997	0.9976	0.99011	0.97138	0.93378	0.86916	0.77067	0.63539	0.46757	0.28261
26												
27												
28	HSENS binomial											
29	X	15	30	45	60	75	90	105	120	135	150	165
30	1	0.46632	0.71519	0.848	0.91888	0.95671	0.9769	0.98767	0.99342	0.99649	0.99813	0.999
31	2	0.12408	0.34989	0.55558	0.7108	0.8179	0.888	0.93232	0.95966	0.97622	0.98611	0.99194
32	3	0.02166	0.12344	0.28053	0.44837	0.59832	0.71888	0.80927	0.87379	0.91816	0.94783	0.96721
33	4	0.00268	0.03308	0.11199	0.23145	0.36989	0.50678	0.62866	0.72938	0.80812	0.86709	0.90975
34	5	0.00025	0.007	0.03633	0.0993	0.1941	0.30956	0.43175	0.5488	0.65288	0.74024	0.81027
35												
36	HSPEC binomial											
37	X	15	30	45	60	75	90	105	120	135	150	165
38	1	0.63325	0.40101	0.25394	0.16081	0.10183	0.06448	0.04083	0.02586	0.01638	0.01037	0.00657
39	2	0.92703	0.77308	0.60736	0.45921	0.33804	0.24398	0.17344	0.12183	0.08475	0.05848	0.04008
40	3	0.99063	0.93993	0.84783	0.73147	0.60833	0.49101	0.38671	0.29844	0.22642	0.16932	0.12506
41	4	0.99915	0.9881	0.95443	0.89426	0.81175	0.71513	0.61317	0.51328	0.42067	0.33844	0.26787
42	5	0.99994	0.99815	0.98905	0.966	0.925	0.86588	0.79177	0.70763	0.61893	0.53066	0.44674

Fig. 8. Spreadsheet (A) and graphic (B) models of the binomial and hypergeometric probability that a diseased herd (HSENS) or nondiseased herd (HSPEC) would be classified correctly based on tests of a sample of individual cattle, assuming that tests were 25% sensitive, 97% specific, that at least 5% of the herd would be infected, and that one positive test result would classify the herd as infected. The positive (HPV+) and negative (HPV−) predictive value of the herd's classification is shown (C), as is the apparent prevalence of diseased herds (HAP), and percent of herds classified correctly (HEFFIC, D) if the true prevalence of infected herds (HP$_D$) was 22%. Part B: diamond = HSENS; triangle = HSPEC; solid line = hypgeom; dotted line = binomial. Part C: diamond = HPV+; triangle = HPV−. Part D: diamond = HEFFIC; triangle = HAP; heavy line = HPD.

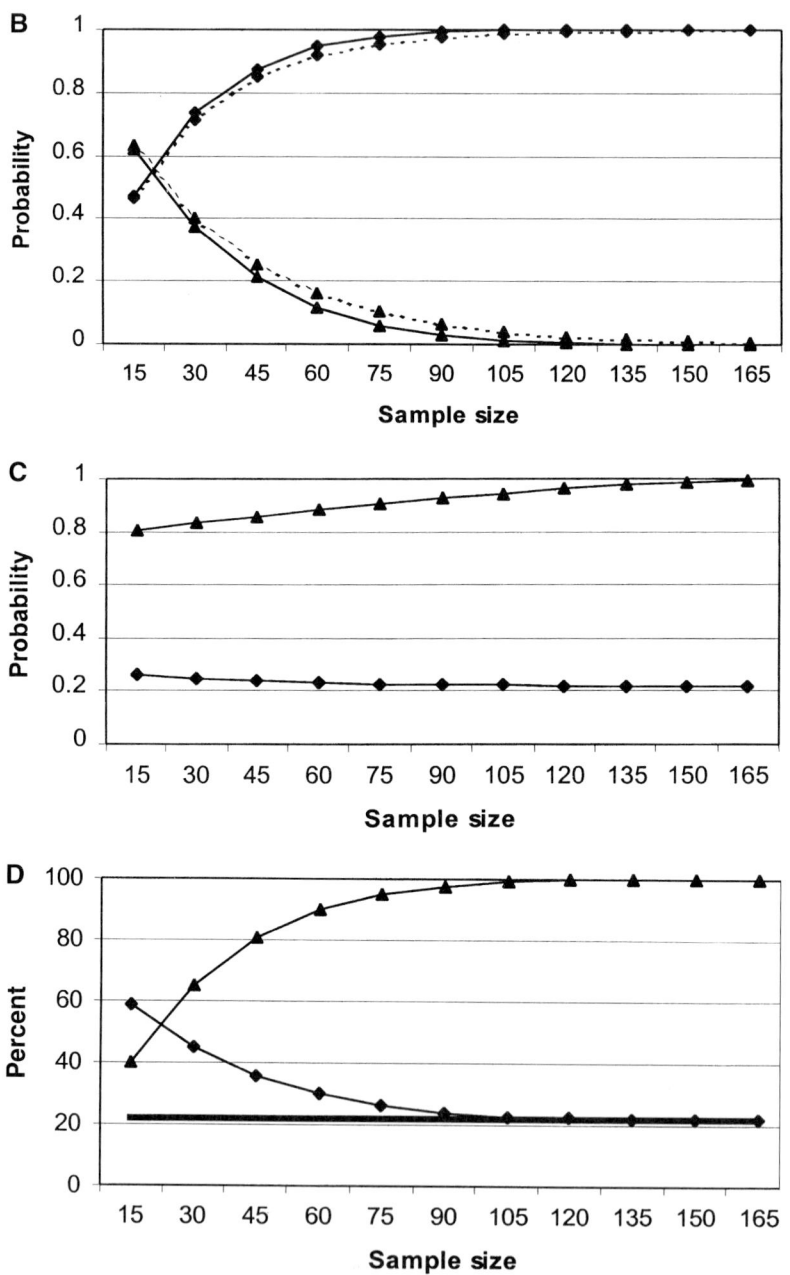

Fig. 8 (continued)

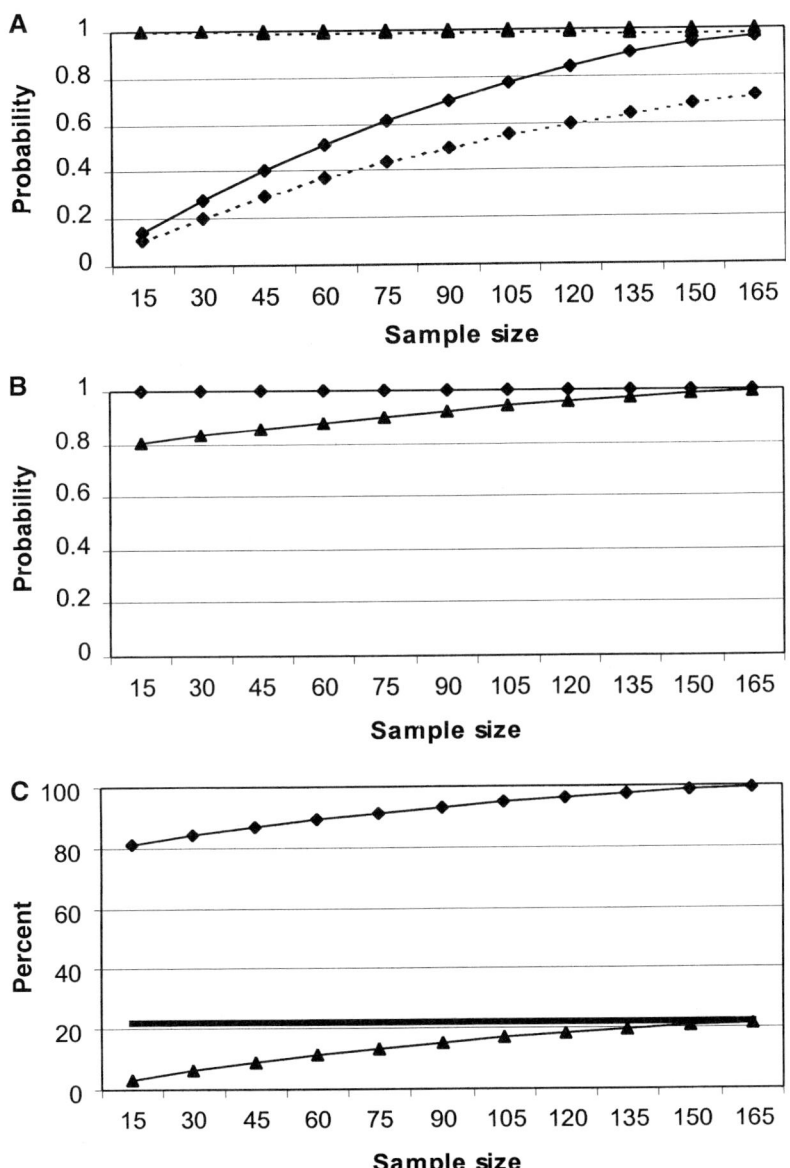

Fig. 9. Graphic model (A) of the binomial and hypergeometric probability that a diseased herd (HSENS) or nondiseased herd (HSPEC) would be classified correctly based on serial testing a sample of individual cattle, assuming that testing was overall 15% sensitive, 99.99% specific, that at least 5% of the herd would be infected, and that one positive test result would classify the herd as infected. The positive (HPV+) and negative (HPV−) predictive value of the herd's classification is shown (B), as is the apparent prevalence of diseased herds (HAP), and percent of herds classified correctly (HEFFIC, C) if the true prevalence of infected herds (HP$_D$) was 22%. Part A: diamond = HSENS; triangle = HSPEC; solid line = hypgeom; dotted line = binomial. Part B: diamond = HPV+; triangle = HPV−. Part C: diamond = HEFFIC; triangle = HAP; heavy line = HPD.

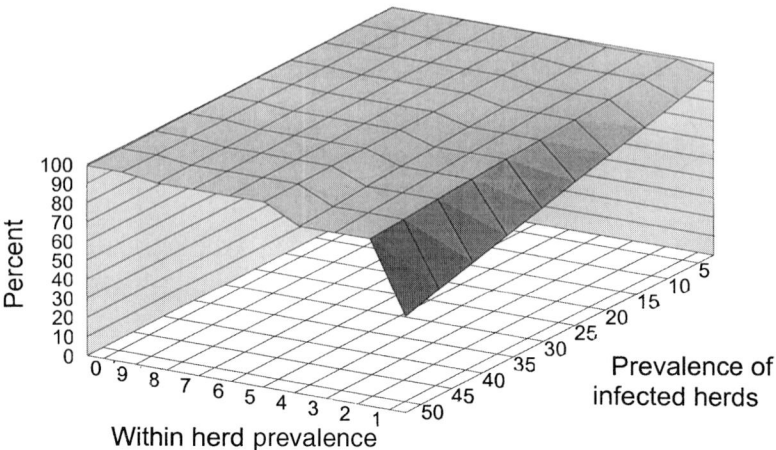

Fig. 10. A three-dimensional graphic model of the percent of herds classified correctly in subpopulations, with a range of within-herd prevalence of infection and with varying prevalence of diseased herds. The model is based on the assumption that 150 cattle were tested from herds of 200, with overall test performance of 15% sensitivity, 99.99% specificity, and that one reactor would classify the herd as diseased.

classification will differ in different-sized herds and in subpopulations in which disease is expected to cluster differently [13].

Summary

Quantitative models simplify reality, and therefore may misrepresent it. With that caution, models can be useful for predicting the outcomes of a variety of what-if scenarios related to biosecurity and biocontainment. Graphic representations of the models help to visualize relationships between factors that influence biosecurity that might not be obvious otherwise. The examples in this article illustrate only a few of many epidemiologic relationships relevant to biosecurity and biocontainment. Many other relationships remain to be explored.

References

[1] Bulagra LL. U.S. voluntary Johne's disease herd status program for cattle. Proceedings of the US Animal Health Association. Richmond (VA): Pat Campbell and Associates and Carter Printing Co.; 1998. p. 420–33.
[2] Byrd DM, Cothern R. Functions, models, and uncertainties. In: Introduction to risk analysis, 1st edition. Rockville (MD): Government Institutes; 2000. p. 41–96.
[3] Byrd DM, Cothern R. Risk analysis. In: Introduction to risk analysis, 1st edition. Rockville (MD): Government Institutes; 2000. p. 1–39.

[4] Daniel WW. Probability distributions. In: Wiley B, editor. Biostatistics: a foundation for analysis in the health sciences, 6th edition. New York: John Wiley & Sons; 1995. p. 79–117.

[5] Dargatz DA, Byrum BA, Barber LK, Sweeney RW, Whitlock RH, Shulah WP, et al. Evaluation of a commercial ELISA for diagnosis of paratuberculosis in cattle. J Am Vet Med Assoc 2001;218:1163–6.

[6] Eppen GD, Gould FJ, Schmidt CP, Moore JH, Weatherford LR. Models and modeling. In: Tucker T, Rifkin S, Evancie K, editors. Introductory management science, 5th edition. Upper Saddle River (NJ): Prentice Hall; 1998. p. 1–27.

[7] Johnson-Ifearulundu Y, Kaneene JB. Distribution and environmental risk factors for paratuberculosis in dairy cattle herds in Michigan. Am J Vet Res 1999;60:589–96.

[8] Jordan D. Aggregate testing for the evaluation of Johne's disease herd status. Aust Vet J 1996;73:16–9.

[9] Jordan D, McEwen SA. Herd-level test performance based on uncertain estimates of individual test performance, individual true prevalence, and herd true prevalence. Prev Vet Med 1998;36:187–209.

[10] Kelling CL, Grotelueschen DM, Smith DR, et al. Testing and management strategies for effective beef and dairy herd BVDV biosecurity programs. The Bovine Practitioner 2000;34: 13–22.

[11] Martin SW. Estimating disease prevalence and the interpretation of screening test results. Prev Vet Med 1984;2:463–72.

[12] Martin SW. The evaluation of tests. Can J Comp Med 1977;41:19–25.

[13] Martin SW, Shoukri M, Thorburn MA. Evaluating the health status of herds based on tests applied to individuals. Prev Vet Med 1992;14:33–43.

[14] McClurkin AW, Littledike ET, Cutlip RC, et al. Production of cattle immunotolerant to bovine viral diarrhea virus. Can J Comp Med 1984;48:156–61.

[15] National Animal Health Monitoring System. Johne's disease on U.S. dairy operations. Publication no. N245.1097. Fort Collins (CO): US Department of Agriculture: Animal and Plant Health Inspection Service: Veterinary Services, Centers for Epidemiology and Animal Health, National Animal Health Monitoring System, 1997. p. 14–27.

[16] Sanderson MW, Dargatz DA, Garry FB. Biosecurity practices of beef cow-calf producers. J Am Vet Med Assoc 2000;217:185–9.

[17] Sterman JD. A skeptic's guide to computer models. In: Barney GO, Kreutzer WB, Garrett MJ, et al., editors. Managing a nation: the microcomputer software catalog, 2nd edition. Boulder (CO): Westview Press; 1991. p. 209–29.

[18] Trajstman AC. Diagnostic tests, sensitivity, specificity, efficiency and prevalence. Aust Vet J 1979;55:501.

[19] Wells SJ. Biosecurity on dairy operations: hazards and risks. J Dairy Sci 2000;83:2380–6.

[20] Winston WL. What is simulation? In: Hinrichs C, Hill J, editors. Simulation modeling using @ Risk. Pacific Grove (CA): Duxbury; 2001. p. 1–7.

[21] Zar JH. More on dichotomous variables. In: Ryu T, Snavely SL, editors. Biostatistical analysis, 4th edition. Upper Saddle River (NJ): Prentice Hall; 1999. p. 516–70.

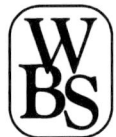

THE VETERINARY
CLINICS
Food Animal
Practice

Vet Clin Food Anim 18 (2002) 177–196

Protecting US cattle
The role of national biosecurity programs

William D. Hueston, DVM, PhD[a],*, Jared D. Taylor[b]

[a]Center for Animal Health and Food Safety, College of Veterinary Medicine,
University of Minnesota, 1365 Gortner Avenue, St. Paul, MN 55108-1016 USA
[b]Virginia-Maryland Regional College of Veterinary Medicine, Blacksburg, VA

The importance of biosecurity in protecting animal agriculture and the food supply received renewed attention because of recent global animal health disasters and the threat of bioterrorism. Bovine spongiform encephalopathy (BSE), first identified in Great Britain in 1986, has swept through Europe. Foot-and-mouth disease (FMD) epidemics have devastated animal industries and disrupted international trade in areas where FMD had previously been contained, including Taiwan, Europe, and much of South America. Bioterrorism galvanized national attention after anthrax spores were distributed through the mail in October of 2001, killing five individuals in the United States and potentially exposing thousands. Although the United States has never identified BSE in native US cattle and has not had an FMD outbreak since 1929, the globalization of animal agriculture and the willingness of terrorists to use zoonoses as biologic weapons have made past successes less predictive of the future. Global commerce and international travel are increasing, so the movement of animals and the diseases that affect them is easier, less expensive, and faster than ever. Many experts say that the question is not "if" but "when" FMD or some other exotic disease will reach the United States, either by accident or by intention. In response, some public figures have demanded that US borders be closed to cattle imports or that the country of origin be conspicuously labeled on imported animal products. Our animal agriculture and food systems are global in nature, however, and country-of-origin labeling is attacked as an infringement on free trade. The veterinary profession stands in the midst of this debate. How well do practicing veterinarians understand the entire biosecurity system of the United States? Can they explain to others what the federal and

---

* Corresponding author.
E-mail address: huest001@umn.edu (W.D. Hueston).

state governments are doing to prevent the introduction of these catastrophic diseases and minimize losses from endemic diseases? Do they know their own professional responsibilities as part of the national biosecurity system?

This article provides insights into the role that practitioners play in national biosecurity and serves as a reference for the most frequently asked questions about the federal role in protection of US animal agriculture. Additionally, it can provide an appreciation of the challenges involved in safeguarding our food supply, animal agriculture, and lifestyle from the animal health threats present around the world.

What is national biosecurity?

Biosecurity involves plans or measures designed to protect populations from transmissible infectious diseases [1]. In common usage, biosecurity also includes the reduction of risks and dangers from predators, invasive species, disease vectors, and potential toxicants, both natural and manmade. National biosecurity, by extension, refers to actions taken to protect the entire population of the nation. Biosecurity can be applied at all levels of production, from the individual farm to corporate policy, from national regulations to international treaties. The levels at which a given disease is addressed typically depend on its prevalence and geographic distribution, direct and indirect economic effect, routes and efficiency of transmission, and available control measures. The impact of diseases must be assessed not only in cattle morbidity and mortality but also in terms of their socioeconomic effects on the nation, including international trade. Generally, to become the focus of national exclusion, control, or eradication, a disease must involve a zoonosis posing an imminent threat to human health or an animal disease that can cause major economic damage to the nation's agriculture and trade. Sufficient technical knowledge and capability must exist to institute appropriate and effective national biosecurity programs. To be effective, producers, agribusiness, consumers, and government agencies must be willing to implement and pay for the prevention and control measures necessary to ensure success.

Recognition of the importance of national biosecurity is not new. The spread of rinderpest across Europe in the mid-1800s led the British to demand trade restrictions to protect Britain's cattle population [2]. Another European rinderpest epidemic just after World War I led to the establishment of the Office International des Epizooties (OIE), the animal health equivalent of the World Health Organization [3]. The OIE advises national veterinary authorities on appropriate measures for preventing the spread of disease through trade in animals and animal products. The OIE currently has more than 140 member countries. OIE recommendations are recognized by the World Trade Organization as the scientific standards for national biosecurity.

The OIE has compiled lists of the animal diseases of greatest public health consequence and socioeconomic impact [4]. These two lists, A and B, are differentiated by the potential for rapid disease spread and the urgency of reporting outbreaks. In theory, list A diseases include those devastating animal diseases with the greatest risk for crossing national borders, such as FMD and rinderpest; however, the decision to categorize a disease is reached by a vote of all of the member countries. The relative importance of individual animal diseases depends, in part, on the animal agriculture of each member country and its domestic experience with the disease. Differences in opinion exist on some diseases that currently appear on list A, such as vesicular stomatitis. The United States has argued that vesicular stomatitis is not a major disease threat to either humans or animals, and therefore, it should be moved to list B. Other countries, however, especially those free of vesicular diseases, consider vesicular stomatitis one of the differentials for FMD and want it left on list A. Bluetongue is another disease for which its importance depends in part on the relative contributions of sheep and goats to the animal agriculture of a country. The US status of OIE list A and B diseases is provided in Tables 1 and 2. These diseases are the primary focus of US national biosecurity programs.

Disease reporting is one of the major functions of the OIE. Prompt dissemination of information on new disease outbreaks and changes in the disease status of regions or countries is critical to successful implementation of appropriate exclusion activities. The signatory countries of the OIE have pledged to report the first occurrence or reoccurrence of list A diseases or any other exceptional epidemiology event within 24 hours by telegram, fax, or e-mail. The OIE then notifies all of the member countries around the world of this new

Table 1
Cattle diseases exotic to the United States

Diseases[a]	Date eradicated/last reported outbreak in the United States
List A	
Foot and mouth	1929
Rinderpest	Never reported
Contagious bovine pleuropneumonia	1892
Lumpy skin disease	Never reported
Rift Valley fever	Never reported
List B	
Bovine babesiosis	1943
Heartwater	Never reported
New World screwworm	Eradicated
Old World screwworm	Never reported
Theileriasis	Never reported
Trypanosomiasis (tsetse transmitted)	Never reported
Bovine spongiform encephalopathy	Never reported

[a] As defined by the Office International des Epizooties.

Table 2
Cattle diseases endemic or sporadic in the United States [DS3]

Diseases[a]	Status[b]	Control programs
List A		
Vesicular stomatitis	Sporadic/regionalized	None
Bluetongue	Sporadic/regionalized	None
List B		
Anthrax	Sporadic/regionalized	None
Pseudorabies	Endemic, regionalized	Eradication
Echinococcosis/hydatidosis	Endemic, uncommon	None
Leptospirosis	Endemic	None
Rabies	Endemic	None
Paratuberculosis	Endemic	None
Trichomoniasis	Endemic	None
Anaplasmosis	Endemic, regionalized	None
Bovine brucellosis	Endemic, regionalized	Eradication
Bovine genital campylobacteriosis	Endemic	None
Bovine tuberculosis	Regionalized	Eradication
Bovine cysticercosis	Endemic	None
Dermatophilosis	Regionalized	None
Enzootic bovine leukosis	Endemic	None
Hemorrhagic septicemia	Sporadic	None
Infectious bovine rhinotracheitis/ infectious pustular vulvovaginitis	Endemic	None
Malignant catarrhal fever	Sporadic	None

[a] As defined by the Office International des Epizooties.

[b] Status descriptions: Sporadic—not occurring every year; endemic—occurring every year; regionalized—limited geographic distribution in U.S.; uncommon—rare diagnoses.

Note: Control program descriptions refer to national biosecurity initiatives only and do not include some state programs.

information. Updates on the status of these new disease occurrences or re-occurrences and any other animal disease information of exceptional importance are communicated internationally through weekly disease information bulletins that are now available through the worldwide Web [5].

National biosecurity efforts have different aims, depending on the specific disease. One goal of national biosecurity is the continued exclusion of diseases. Exclusion targets include diseases that are exotic to the nation, the so-called foreign animal diseases (see Table 1), and the diseases for which national control or eradication programs exist. Other national biosecurity measures are directed at endemic diseases, and thus may be more appropriately termed *biocontainment*. Biocontainment programs seek to prevent further spread of specific diseases from limited geographic areas, although their ultimate goal may be complete eradication. This distinction between biosecurity activities directed toward exclusion and biocontainment activities including control and eradication is an arbitrary dichotomy used throughout this article. All national biosecurity programs are interrelated, where expenditures and challenges vary over time, as the priorities for exclusion, control, and eradication change.

The United States has a successful history of national biosecurity programs. Contagious bovine pleuropneumonia, FMD, babesiosis, and screwworm have been eradicated. Bovine tuberculosis and brucellosis are under control and close to eradication. The foreign animal disease exclusion efforts also have been successful to date, but continued success is complicated by the fact that these diseases (and many others) are present in many regions of the world. Expansion of global commerce and travel and the demonstrated potential for bioterrorism increase the threat of exotic disease introduction into the United States.

National biosecurity exclusion activities

Disease introduction can occur through human or animal activity, intentionally or accidentally (Table 3). Consequently, a series of risk mitigation and interdiction measures exist to prevent entry through the importation, smuggling, or trans-shipment of animals and animal byproducts. Exclusion of diseases from the United States begins in the exporting country, with specific prohibitions, health certifications, pre-export testing, and quarantine. The US Department of Agriculture, Animal and Plant Health Inspection Service's (APHIS) International Services has personnel stationed around the

Table 3
Potential source of disease exposure

Disease	Live cattle	Other animals	Germplasm	Animal products	Vectors	Fomites	Humans
Highest risk diseases							
Foot and mouth	+++	+++	++	+++	+	+	+
Bovine spongiform encephalopathy	+++	+	±	+++	–	–	–
Other foreign animal diseases							
Rinderpest	+++	++	+	+	–	+	–
Contagious bovine pleuropneumonia	+++	++	–	+	–	–	–
Lumpy skin disease	+++	++	+	++	–	–	–
Rift Valley	+++	+++	–	–	++	–	+++
Heartwater	+++	++	–	–	–	–	–
Theileriasis	+++	++	–	–	+++	–	–
Screwworm	+++	++	–	–	++	–	+
Trypanosomiasis	+++	++	–	–	+++	–	+

+++ Most effective source of disease exposure.
++ Important source of disease exposure.
+ Less likely source of disease exposure.
± Potential but unproven sources of disease exposure.
– Not recognized as a source of disease exposure.

world to monitor animal disease issues and to work with countries on programs that reduce the risk of disease transmission in trade with the United States. The International Services personnel help establish surveillance programs, create zoning/regionalization plans, and develop programs for pre-export testing (although primary responsibility for implementing these procedures rests with the country of origin). In limited instances, such as Mexico and Central America, International Services has taken an active role collaborating in eradication and exclusion efforts for specific diseases (such as FMD and screwworms throughout Mexico and Central America).

Exclusion activities also cover the means of conveyance of the animals and animal products into the United States, focusing on cleaning and disinfection to preclude exposure during the import shipment. On arrival at the US border, exclusion activities comprise review of documentation and identification, visual inspection, retesting, and quarantine. Prophylactic treatment may be conducted for specific disease agents and vectors, including internal and external parasites. Animals and animal products successfully meeting all import requirements enter US commerce without further restrictions. No requirement exists for permanent identification of all imports as distinct from US-born animals; however, certain classes of cattle may require permanent identification. Mexican-origin cattle destined for feedlots are at greater risk of bovine tuberculosis than US cattle, so these animals are permanently identified to minimize the potential for confusion in the tuberculosis eradication program.

The trans-shipment of animals through the United States represents another potential mechanism for introduction of exotic diseases. Trans-shipment relates to the movement of animals from another country through US territory en route to export through a US port. Specific protocols must be developed regarding trans-shipped animals in the same manner that import protocols are negotiated.

Import requirements are developed on the basis of the disease status of the countries of origin and destination and the characteristics of the proposed animal and animal product import. Generic trade guidelines are published by the OIE as the International Animal Health Code [4]. The code is recognized as the international standard by the World Trade Organization and cannot be challenged in world courts. Countries may require import health requirements in excess of the code recommendations, so long as they are science-based and justified through risk analysis as agreed in the sanitary/phytosanitary provisions of the General Agreement on Tariffs and Trade during the Uruguay round [6]. Import restrictions in excess of OIE Code recommendations also are subject to arbitration through the World Trade Organization. The US Department of Agriculture, through the APHIS's Veterinary Services (VS), negotiates import protocols on a country-by-country basis. Import permits prepared by VS specify the animals or products to be imported and refer to the required testing, health certifications, and quarantine outlined in the import protocol.

The Uruguay round of the General Agreement on Tariffs and Trade also formalized the concept of regionalization. Because diseases do not recognize national borders, the World Trade Organization now recognizes that geographic boundaries may serve as a better demarcation of health status than political subdivisions. The trade agreement specifically acknowledges geographic zones within a country or regions encompassing multiple countries as legitimate components of trade agreements. A negotiated import protocol may allow entry of animals from a free zone within an otherwise infected country, so long as the two countries can agree on the area within the zone and the regulatory conditions necessary to guarantee that the zone is indeed free of the disease and that the animal actually originated from that zone.

Table 3 divides the most important cattle diseases into two major risk categories. Risk involves both the likelihood of disease introduction and the consequences if the disease were to become established. Two diseases are listed in the highest-risk category, FMD and BSE. FMD is considered to be the most highly contagious animal pathogen known. Although FMD has been successfully excluded from the United States since 1929, the costs of its introduction would be enormous in terms of stamping out the outbreak and the negative effects on US agricultural trade. BSE is not considered a contagious disease, but its long incubation period, unremarkable clinical signs, and difficulties of recognition and diagnosis mean that the disease would be difficult to identify and eradicate quickly if found in native US cattle. Diagnosis of BSE in native US cattle would disrupt the entire cattle industry and cripple international trade. Unlike FMD, BSE also has public health implications in terms of variant Creutzfeldt-Jakob disease.

The entire US network of exclusion controls can be illustrated through an examination of the risks associated with importation of live cattle, cattle products, and germplasm (semen and embryos). Controls on animals other than cattle, animal products, and other agricultural goods that pose a risk of introducing cattle disease agents or vectors also are discussed. The authors examine threats associated with human travel, illegal smuggling of potentially dangerous material, and intentional exposure (terrorism).

Live cattle imports

Table 3 demonstrates that affected live cattle represent the most effective source of exposure for most of the foreign animal diseases. Consequently, greater restrictions generally are placed on live animal imports than on germplasm, products, or people. As a result of the strict restrictions on live cattle and other animals, animal products may represent the most likely route of introduction of foreign animal diseases into the United States because of the volume of trade and the wide dissemination throughout the country.

Ensuring the health and safety of imports begins at the country of origin. This undertaking involves a coordinated effort between the owners of the animals or products, the exporter (and importer), the recognized veterinary authority of the country of origin, and the US Department of Agriculture, APHIS, VS. The US exclusion efforts and OIE recommendations were designed principally to prevent the introduction of FMD and rinderpest, the two most highly contagious cattle diseases (the classic cattle plagues). Current US regulations forbid the direct importation of ruminants from countries in which FMD, rinderpest, and BSE are present [7]. Importation of animals from these countries requires quarantine and testing to ensure their freedom from these diseases before entry to the United States.

Individual animal testing requirements are negotiated on a country-by-country basis. If a potential exporting country claims to be free of a disease exotic to the United States, that claim must be certified by a team of US Department of Agriculture inspectors. Before leaving the country of origin, all animals destined for export must be free of any clinical signs of illness based on a thorough physical examination by an officially recognized veterinarian, typically an employee of the government of the country of origin. The animal also must have an acceptable means of identification. The animal identification and certification of health status are recorded on an export health certificate, along with an assurance that the animals meet all of the testing requirements of the negotiated import protocol.

The United States imports the largest number of cattle from its two neighbors, Mexico and Canada. The US Department of Agriculture, APHIS, VS recorded 2,260,378 imported cattle during calendar year 2000, 99% of which originated from Canada and Mexico [8]. The United States collaborates with these two countries to achieve a similar level of animal health throughout all of North America as a result of the North American Free Trade Agreement. The chief veterinary officials of the United States, Mexico, and Canada meet on a regular basis to ensure continual communication and to strengthen joint animal health initiatives. Cattle coming from Mexico and Canada require documentation similar to that necessary for interstate movement within the United States (e.g., tested for tuberculosis or from a certified free herd; tested or vaccinated for brucellosis; and no apparent signs of any illness or disease). Additionally, cattle coming from regions of Mexico infested with cattle fever ticks must be dipped with an approved acaricide before submission for import and are dipped again at the border inspection station.

More extensive documentation or testing must be performed on animals from other countries for diseases exotic to the United States. Testing also is required for endemic diseases for which the United States has control and eradication programs, such as brucellosis and tuberculosis. Because some diseases are transmitted by insect vectors, imported cattle must be properly treated for parasites (typically with an avermectin) before importation. An import permit and a copy of all negative test results, inspection certificates, and identification must accompany animals throughout the import process. Once they arrive in the United States, all cattle from countries other than Mexico and Canada are quarantined at an official US Department of

Agriculture facility for 30 days, and necessary testing is repeated for all diseases of importance. If any animal tests positive for a disease while in quarantine, it will be refused entry into the United States or destroyed. Depending on the disease, the entire shipment and any animals that contacted the affected animal may be refused or destroyed (David Vogt, DVM, US Department of Agriculture:APHIS:VS, personal communication, May 2001). The importation process is time consuming and expensive; consequently, only a limited number of live animals are brought into the United States.

Germplasm

The stringent policies on live cattle imports have led many of those who want to import genetics to turn to semen and embryo importation. In these cases, the donors of the imported germplasm are tested and certified, similar to standards used for live animal imports. Embryos and semen can even be imported from nations with FMD, provided certain conditions are met. First, donors must not have been vaccinated against FMD, nor can they come from or be housed or collected in a region affected by an outbreak in the previous year. Second, the semen and embryo collection and handling practices must conform to OIE standards and must be observed by personnel from the US Department of Agriculture, APHIS, VS. These biosecurity protections facilitate the use of embryos and semen as a safe, economical, and effective way to share genetics internationally, with minimal risk from foreign animal diseases. Internationally accepted procedures for safe collection of bovine embryos are outlined in *The Manual of the International Embryo Transfer Society* [9]. Disease-specific standards for movement of both semen and embryos are found in the OIE International Animal Health Code [4]. A total of 1266 embryos and 2,693,158 straws of semen were imported in the United States in 2000, originating from a total of 14 countries. Canada was the source of the largest number of imports (94.5% of embryos and 81.7% of semen) [8].

Import of animals other than cattle

Many list A and B cattle diseases also can affect other species; therefore, to protect cattle, import of other species is subject to restrictions similar to those imposed on cattle. Interest in importing both domestic and wild animals may be driven by a variety of interests. Bush-tail possums from New Zealand received a short flurry of attention as exotic pets until their role as a reservoir for bovine tuberculosis was recognized and the trade was prohibited.

Some species of animals may serve as mechanical vectors for cattle disease, even though they themselves are not affected. For example, although horses are not susceptible to FMD, they must not have been in areas infected with FMD nor been in contact with animals that have been in an FMD-affected area within the 5 days prior to shipping for fear that they may contribute to the spread of this extremely contagious disease.

Risk from importation of nonbovine animals also originates from their ability to harbor vectors, which in turn can introduce a cattle disease. For example, *Cowdria ruminantium*, the rickettsial agent of heartwater, is transmitted by ticks (principally *Amblyomma* genus). Although heartwater is not present in the United States, potential vectors are. If the disease were introduced, it would be difficult to eliminate. In 1998 and 1999, African spurred tortoises and leopard tortoises imported through Florida ports were found to be infested with ticks carrying *C. ruminantium*. This incident led the Florida Fish and Wildlife Conservation Agency to establish an emergency prohibition of the importation of African spurred and leopard tortoises in late 1999. This exclusion was broadened by the US Department of Agriculture, APHIS, VS in 2000 to prohibit import or interstate transportation of either tortoise, and the ban was extended to include the Bell's hingeback tortoise. Although such issues garner far less attention than FMD, they are still significant to national biosecurity and the protection of American agriculture.

Animal and agricultural products

Examination of past outbreaks suggests that animal products represent the most common vehicle for dissemination of both FMD and BSE, but they are less important for rinderpest and pleuropneumonia and play no role in the introduction of vector-borne diseases. Pre-export testing and treatments, health certification, and postentry quarantine create multiple barriers that mitigate the risk of entry of foreign animal diseases through live cattle and other animals. As a result, the most effective source for exotic disease exposure, the live animal import, is not the most likely scenario for a foreign animal disease outbreak. From a risk perspective, animal products represent a much more likely scenario for introduction of exotic diseases or pests because of the magnitude of trade, the difficulty of assessing the health risks associated with bulk shipments, and the lack of permanent, unalterable identification of the source and composition of these products.

Animal products can introduce diseases almost as effectively as live animals. Contaminated clothing, equipment, and bedding also can harbor disease agents. Consequently, import protocols have been developed for other agricultural products and materials with potential contact with animal disease agents or vectors. These protocols consider the processing techniques for the imported goods along with the survival characteristics of the specific pathogens and vectors. For example, the FMD agent is quite sensitive to temperature and pH changes, so pork products such as hams that have been cooked or cured sufficiently to inactivate the FMD virus may be imported from FMD-infected countries. Processing requirements have been developed for a wide range of products, including hides, hoofs and horns, feedstuffs, and manure. Products arriving at US ports of entry without proper documentation or evidence of the required processing must undergo disinfection and be returned to the country of origin, or they are destroyed. Disposition of intercepted products depends on the product, the disease status of the country of origin, and the ability of the importer and exporter to meet the costs.

Similar risks exist for garbage originating abroad. Food waste from ships, airplanes, or international arrivals has been incriminated in many exotic disease outbreaks. Consequently, regulations require that such waste be stored in leak-proof, sealed containers during transport and disposed of through incineration, sterilization, or other processes approved by the US Department of Agriculture.

Human travel

International travel takes place frequently. An estimated 400,000,000 international travelers entered the United States in 1999 by airplane, boat, train, bus, foot, and private vehicles [10]. Table 3 illustrates that humans and fomites (such as shoes) represent a less likely source of disease exposure; however, given the huge number of international visitors and the attention focused on excluding high-risk cattle and animal products, less likely means of disease spread may represent a larger proportion of the overall national risk. The US Department of Agriculture, APHIS Plant Protection and Quarantine works closely with US Customs Service to ensure a strong presence at international airports, seaports, and border stations. The Plant Protection and Quarantine inspectors check passengers, baggage, cargo, and international mail packages for products that may harbor animal or plant pests or disease organisms. All international travelers are required to complete a Customs Declaration, disclosing all products or goods brought into the United States. One question on the form relates directly to animal health issues. All persons entering the United States are required to respond "yes" or "no" to the following question: "I am (We are) bringing fruits, plants, meats, food, soil, birds, snails, other live animals, wildlife products, farm products; or, have been on a farm or ranch outside the U.S." [11].

Dogs trained to detect the scents of animal and plant products also are used by APHIS to screen passengers, their luggage, carry-on baggage, and mail packages from abroad. The "Beagle Brigade" represents a visible and popular component of the national biosecurity program related to returning travelers and visitors to the United States.

Certain highly contagious agents, including FMD and rinderpest, can remain infective for a significant length of time in association with nonanimal organic material such as dirt. Port inspectors therefore also examine footwear from travelers arriving from infected countries. Soiled footwear is disinfected before entering the United States.

The heightened awareness of biosecurity in the wake of the UK FMD experience in the spring of 2001 led to increased efforts to inform travelers of the potential risks. Extra educational efforts were directed at returning international travelers to increase voluntary declaration of forbidden materials, and voluntary initiatives were encouraged. US travelers returning from affected countries are encouraged to avoid farms, sale barns, stockyards, animal laboratories, packing houses, zoos, fairs, or other animal facilities for 5 days after returning to the United States. These exhortations are disseminated through the lay press, leaflets, and signs at locations where the public is most likely to come into contact with animals, such as fairs, horse shows, or zoos.

Unintentional and intentional introduction of exotic disease agents into the United States

APHIS reported approximately 300,000 interceptions of meat, poultry, and animal byproducts at international border ports and through inspection of international mail in 1998 [10]. Most of these potential introductions seem to have been accidental, rather than intentional. Nevertheless, the sheer volume of international travel and trade can overwhelm the exclusion system. Intentional smuggling of prohibited materials does occur, primarily for commercial reasons.

The World Trade Center attack of September 2001 and the anthrax dispersal through the mail in October of that year focused attention on the potential for bioterrorism and its corollary, agroterrorism. Many of the biologic agents considered by the Centers for Disease Control and Prevention to be the most likely weapons of bioterrorism are zoonotic diseases such as anthrax, plague, and tularemia, all three of which occur naturally in the United States. The most worrisome potential agents for agroterrorism, however, are exotic to the United States, including FMD, rinderpest, and Rift Valley fever. Agroterrorists most likely target agriculture to disrupt the economy, although creating public hysteria concerning the safety of the food supply may be a secondary goal.

Emergency response

No exclusion system is perfect, so no "zero risk" exists for the introduction of exotic diseases. Whether accidental or intentional, foreign animal disease introduction will occur in the United States. When exclusion measures fail to prevent entry of a foreign animal disease, national biosecurity relies on rapid detection and prompt emergency response.

Cattle owners and private practitioners are the first line of defense for detection of exotic diseases, by diagnostic scrutiny of ill animals. Prompt diagnostic work-up is important in the event of unusual disease occurrences such as the appearance of vesicular lesions or high morbidity and mortality in herds. State and federal veterinary officials provide no-cost diagnostic consultation in these circumstances to help rule out potential foreign animal diseases. Specially trained state and federal foreign animal disease diagnosticians are stationed throughout the country. These veterinarians have witnessed clinical cases of exotic diseases of concern to the United States and are trained in case-finding and diagnostic sample collection to support emergency response. Testing and diagnostics are performed at no charge to the producer or veterinarian by authorized state or federal laboratories. If a list A disease is suspected, immediate actions may be initiated before laboratory confirmation. Quarantines can be applied to affected facilities or farms and potentially to the surrounding area, depending on the circumstances. Restrictions on movement apply to all livestock and animals, and movement of equipment, vehicles, or personnel requires proper sanitation measures. Trace-back would begin immediately to locate animals, people, or vehicles that have contacted the suspect property. An assessment as to whether wild animals may be a risk factor in the dissemination or persistence of infection also would be needed, and additional actions would be taken to address this potential threat.

If the diagnosis of an OIE list A disease is confirmed, more extensive measures would be instituted by state and federal veterinary authorities. The actions taken depend on the agent and the specific details of the case; however, a state of emergency would likely be proclaimed, either by the state or federal government. This declaration authorizes quarantine, seizure, and disposal of potentially affected or exposed animals. The producers and state and federal officials determine the fair market value of destroyed livestock, and producers are reimbursed 100%. The cost of indemnity is shared equally by the state and federal governments, although the federal government may pay more than 50% if a state does not have adequate matching funds. Producers who intentionally move or handle animals in a manner that violates the law receive no payment for destroyed animals and may face legal charges.

Early detection is critical to ensure that the disease does not spread beyond the first-affected premise. Because most foreign animal diseases can be transmitted by both direct and indirect contact, zones of protection are usually demarcated around infected areas. In the case of FMD, susceptible animals are eliminated within the zone. Vaccination may be a viable option for some diseases with widespread incursions, but vaccination itself carries some risks. The immune response to the vaccines for several foreign animal diseases, such as FMD, is indistinguishable from that of the disease itself. Because some affected animals can be asymptomatic carriers of the disease or can shed for significant lengths of time after abatement of signs, positive serology suggests the risk of the disease. Vaccinated animals must be destroyed eventually, therefore, along with naturally exposed animals to re-establish disease freedom for the country. As a result, countries that are free of those diseases can refuse entry of any animals in which vaccination has been practiced (in the case of FMD, up to 12 months after vaccination has ceased).

Specific emergency response plans for each of the foreign animal diseases are prepared by APHIS and documented in foreign animal disease Emergency Disease Guidelines. Individual states may supplement these national plans with their own emergency response guidelines. These plans cover prevention and control strategies, treatment or destruction of affected animals, and other logistics. Mock outbreaks are held from time to time as training exercises. These mock exercises help identify weaknesses in the emergency response system. The success of the US exclusion efforts creates one of the greatest challenges for our emergency response capabilities. Without the experience of dealing with real outbreaks, preparedness must rely on education and training. US veterinarians are sent to other countries in which animal health emergencies actually exist to gain the experience needed for preparedness. Government and private practice veterinarians sent to help with the 2001 FMD outbreak in the United Kingdom were provided with invaluable training.

Biocontainment of endemic diseases

National biocontainment programs comprise federally supported disease prevention and control programs. The most visible programs seek to eradicate cattle diseases of serious economic or public health impact, such as brucellosis and tuberculosis. The decision to initiate a national biocontainment program depends on scientific and political factors. The United States does not have biocontainment programs in place for all of the OIE list A and B diseases found within the country (see Table 2). National biocontainment programs can be mandatory, such as for brucellosis and tuberculosis, or voluntary, such as federal guidelines established to recognize anaplasmosis-free herds and paratuberculosis status programs. Voluntary certification programs with government oversight are gaining additional momentum as added value is recognized for the documented animal health and welfare status of herds of origin. Although voluntary certification programs and third-party verification schemes may address customer concerns, most international trading partners insist on federal involvement in export certifications.

Other national biocontainment programs seek to restrict the geographic range of a disease for the purpose of creating disease-free zones. The establishment of disease-free zones within a country has been recognized by the OIE and World Trade Organization as a legitimate approach to facilitating safe trade from countries in which specific diseases are endemic. The United States has used the disease-free zone concept for bluetongue to facilitate exports of semen. Bluetongue zoning depends on both serologic surveillance of cattle and a survey of vector presence and competence for transmitting the virus.

The legal basis of national biosecurity programs

National biosecurity programs, both for exclusion and biocontainment, operate within the legal framework of the US Constitution and the laws and regulations of the nation. The Constitution assigns to the federal government the sole authority to regulate international agreements and interstate commerce. All other rights are retained by the state governments. Except in the case of a declared national emergency, the federal government has limited animal health authorities within each state. Consequently, US national biosecurity programs have evolved as collaborative efforts between the federal and state governments. Most animal health programs at the state level are administered cooperatively, with federal and state veterinary officials sharing the responsibilities for implementation.

Most of the federal government's authority and responsibility for animal health currently resides with the US Department of Agriculture. The US Department of Agriculture was created in 1862. The first US Department of Agriculture head recognized the role of imported animals in the spread of disease and encouraged quarantine of imported animals [12]. Initial legislation requiring import quarantine gave the authority to the Treasury Department; however, this law was never implemented. A federal agency directed toward animal disease control was not established until 1884, with the Bureau of Animal Industry [13]. Interestingly, the legislation was hotly debated as an issue of state's rights, finally passing with a vote of 155 to 127. Disease eradication and subsequent exclusion were the initial priorities of the Bureau of Animal Industry. The first programmatic success of the Bureau of Animal Industry was the eradication of contagious bovine pleuropneumonia in 1892.

Within the US Department of Agriculture, APHIS is the primary agency charged with regulatory rule-making and enforcement of national biosecurity programs. APHIS is divided into operational divisions that implement the regulations in the field: International Services, which performs all APHIS activity outside of the United States; VS, which deals with live animal issues within the United States and issues import permits for live animals, germplasm, and animal byproducts, including animal-derived biologicals and reagents originating abroad; and Plant Protection and Quarantine, which oversees exclusion activities at ports of entry in conjunction with the Treasury Department's Customs Service. Another US Department of Agriculture agency, the Food Safety Inspection Service, is charged with inspection of food products (including meat and poultry) imported into the United States. Research on the highest-risk exotic cattle diseases, such as FMD and rinderpest, is restricted to Plum Island Animal Disease Center. The US Department of Agriculture Agricultural Research Service and APHIS, Veterinary Services share Plum Island for basic and applied research, diagnostics, and training programs concerning the most threatening of the foreign animal diseases. Non-US Department of Agriculture departments involved with biosecurity responsibilities include Health and Human Services and Interior. The Health and Human Services Food and Drug Administration, through the Center for Veterinary Medicine, has authority for some animal products, such as animal feeds. The Interior Department's Fish and Wildlife Service has responsibility for wildlife.

These jurisdictional divisions may seem clear cut; however, in reality, the programmatic responsibility for many issues may not be delineated so easily. Decision making and implementation of biosecurity programs at the federal level typically involve coordination among all of these agencies. The federal government's authority is restricted to international agreements and interstate movement. Almost all biosecurity authorities at the farm level remain within an individual state's rights.

The general program directions and legal authorities for national biosecurity programs are established by congressional legislation. Actual regulations covering the daily program operation are promulgated by government agencies such as APHIS and finalized after opportunity for public comment. Program priorities also can be influenced by the congressional budgeting process, because resources often determine whether individual programs can be implemented successfully. Subsequent to the passage of legislation, the authorized federal agency develops the detailed program guidelines that are promulgated as federal regulations. All legislation and regulation must fall within the Constitutional mandate, with challenges settled in federal courts.

Biosecurity programs at the state level are authorized by state legislation. Individual states may establish state biosecurity programs that exceed those of the national programs; however, states cannot opt out of participation in national programs or set state requirements for testing, vaccination, and control less stringent than federal regulations where they exist. State legislation and regulation may vary widely for those diseases for which no national program exists. The Constitution specifically excludes the right of states to enter into international trade agreements with foreign countries.

A system implemented through cooperation

National biosecurity is achieved through the combined efforts of federal and state governments, agribusiness, and the producers. In promulgating regulations, the concerns of environmental, animal welfare, food safety, and other interest groups are considered. Implementation of this biosecurity system requires collaboration and cooperation on a daily basis. Implementation plans are developed in concert with state governments and the affected agricultural industries. Federal agencies work with state authorities in reporting, monitoring, and testing for specified diseases.

Neither the federal or state veterinary services have sufficient numbers of personnel to implement all of the existing national biosecurity programs. The federal government designed the "accredited veterinarian" program to authorize private veterinary practitioners to act on behalf of the federal government in the implementation of specific regulatory programs. Accredited veterinarians test animals and collect diagnostic samples for national eradication programs, such as those for brucellosis and tuberculosis. Accredited veterinarians also conduct physical examinations of animals intended for interstate movement or international export and complete the certificate of veterinary inspection for federal endorsement. Recently, the federal government has begun to recruit private practice veterinarians to be available on an as-needed basis in the event of the declaration of an extraordinary emergency or some other animal health disaster. State and federal cooperation with producers and local veterinarians is paramount for the success of national biosecurity programs, particularly for endemic diseases.

The bovine practitioner's role in national biosecurity

The bovine practitioner is a key contributor to the national biosecurity system, for both exclusion and biocontainment. Practitioners have greater daily interaction with animal owners and producers than any state or federal veterinary officials. The practitioner is therefore the logical first point of contact if the producer or an employee observes an ill animal or an unusual condition. Understandably, practitioners may feel that they are in an awkward situation when they see animals showing clinical signs such as vesicular lesions around the mouth or coronary band that are compatible with one of the foreign animal diseases. On the one hand, veterinarians remember the old adage "when you hear hoofbeats in the hallway behind you, don't think 'zebra' first." At the same time, the practitioner must guard against complacency, that is, the sense that "it can't happen here." The veterinarian must be aware of the potential for a perceived conflict of interest, because the owner is paying for the services of the veterinarian. The accredited veterinarian completing regulatory program activities as an agent of the government has primary responsibility to the federal government, even though the specific activities are paid for by the animal owner or agent.

Thorough clinical evaluation of ill cattle and careful questioning about the epidemiologic patterns of the disease are critical to the ongoing national biosecurity system. Imported cattle that become ill raise special concerns and need to be evaluated with extra scrutiny to ensure that they are not exhibiting signs of a disease exotic to the United States. Other management and environmental issues must be factored into the evaluation as well, such as any history of foreign travel or visitors and the nutrition and housing of the animals. Understandably, the practitioner does not want to raise undue suspicions by calling in regulatory officials, but the alternative situation may be even worse. Failure to detect a foreign animal disease early in the outbreak compounds the challenges of responding effectively to it. Consultations with state and federal foreign animal disease diagnosticians and the supporting laboratory diagnostic work are provided without charge to the owner or the veterinarian. State and federal regulatory officials need opportunities to join bovine practitioners evaluating field cases to keep their diagnostic skills sharp. Practitioners can take advantage of these work-ups for unusual cases to gain additional diagnostic support, and potentially, on-the-job continuing education.

Bovine practitioners also play a vital role in domestic biocontainment programs. The veterinary accreditation program empowers private veterinary practitioners to act as government officials for the purpose of regulatory programs. Accreditation provides a force of trained professionals to complement state and federal veterinary services. Examining animals, collecting diagnostic samples, interpreting diagnostic results, and completing health papers are critical to the safe movement of animals interstate and internationally.

Bovine practitioners working with purebred cattle producers have additional responsibilities associated with the marketing and movement of animals, semen, and embryos. Producers of purebred herds are more likely to purchase breeding stock or germplasm imported from abroad. The owner needs to be encouraged to ensure that the country of origin and associated health papers remain a part of each import's medical records in the event of illness or the emergence of a new animal disease in the country of origin. Establishing the herd health status and documenting the individual animal or donor's health status require extra attention to animal identification and record keeping. The practitioner becomes part of the team in building the health certification necessary to market and move the animals or germplasm.

The bovine practitioner is an important contributor to the national biosecurity system, ensuring qualified veterinary expertise at the farm level. Good veterinary-client-patient relationships provide the first line of defense against the emergence of new diseases, the spread of endemic diseases, or the outbreak of exotic diseases. Maintaining current knowledge about foreign animal diseases and domestic disease control programs is paramount for every practitioner: "forewarned is forearmed."

Conclusions

The US national biosecurity system is only as strong as its weakest link. No individual component of the system is fail safe; exotic diseases will evade exclusion and enter the country occasionally. New diseases and conditions will continue to emerge in the dynamic interaction among agent, host, and environment. Emerging diseases must be considered the norm rather than the exception.

Prior experience with foreign animal disease exclusion may not be predictive of the future. The 1929 introduction of FMD into the United States was contained successfully with low numbers of animals slaughtered because of early detection and prompt response. Animal agriculture in the United States is dramatically different today, however, and human population increases combined with significant societal changes mean that a new introduction could not be handled in the same manner as in 1929. The experiences of the United Kingdom in responding to FMD in 2001 provide a sobering insight into the myriad challenges created by an exotic disease introduction. By the time it was initially confirmed, the disease was widespread owing to a combination of unlawful and legal activities. Exposed animals had been shipped throughout the country, creating multiple disease foci. Destruction of the affected and exposed animals proved to be a major challenge owing to personnel shortages and bureaucratic delays surrounding environmental permitting for carcass destruction. Even after the military became involved, some social and political issues complicated the emergency response. Consideration of these experiences in the development of emergency preparedness plans and simulated outbreaks can help the United States become better prepared.

The bovine practitioner has a critical role to play in promoting biosecurity at both the farm level and the national level. Successful exclusion of exotic diseases, biocontainment of endemic diseases, and emergency preparedness rest soundly on bovine practitioners as part of the national biosecurity team. Bovine practitioners must voice their opinions on the strengths and weaknesses of existing and proposed national biosecurity programs. Healthy debate about national biosecurity programs and consideration of biosecurity issues by national veterinary organizations provide valuable feedback for the continual improvement of the programs and enhance their credibility. The health and productivity of US agriculture depend on national biosecurity.

References

[1] Toma B, Vallaincourt J-P, Dufour B, Eliot M, Moutou F, Marsh W, et al., editors. Dictionary of veterinary epidemiology. Ames (IA): Iowa State University Press; 1999. p. 24.
[2] Dunlop R, Williams D. Veterinary medicine: an illustrated history. St. Louis: Mosby; 1996. p. 377.
[3] Office International des Epizooties. World Organization for animal health, 75 years, 10th edition. Paris: OIE; 1999. p 13–17.
[4] Office International des Epizooties. International animal health code, Paris: OIE; 2001. Available at: http://www.oie.int/eng/normes/mcode/a_summry.htm. Accessed 3/3/02.
[5] Office International des Epizooties. Disease information. Available at: http://www.oie.int/eng/info/hebdo/a_info.htm. Accessed 3/3/02.
[6] World Trade Organization. Agreement on the application of sanitary and phytosanitary measures (SPS agreement). In: The results of the Uruguay round of multilateral trade negotiations: the legal texts. Geneva, Switzerland; 1994. Available at: http://www.wto.int/english/tratop_e/sps_e/spsagr_e.htm. Accessed 3/3/02.
[7] National Archives and Records Administration. Code of federal regulations: Title 9, animals and animal products. Washington (DC), 2001. Available at: http://www.access.gpo.gov/nara/cfr/waisidx_01/9cfrvl_01.html. Accessed 3/3/02.
[8] United States Department of Agriculture. Animal and Plant Health Inspection Service, Veterinary Services, Center for Animal Disease Information Analysis. Import tracking system. Ft. Collins (CO), 2001.
[9] Stringfellow D, Seidel G. editors. The manual of the international embryo transfer society, 3rd edition. Savoy (IL), 1998.
[10] Wilson T, Logan-Henfry L, Weller R, Kellman B. Antiterrorism, biological crimes, and biological warfare targeting animal agriculture. In: Brown C, Bolin C, editors. Emerging diseases of animals. Washington (DC): ASM Press; 2000. p. 44.

[11] United States Department of the Treasury. Customs Service. Customs declaration (customs form 6059B). Washington (DC): US Government Printing Office; 1991.
[12] Dunlop R, Williams D. Veterinary medicine: an illustrated history. St. Louis: Mosby; 1996. p. 417–20.
[13] Dunlop R, Williams D. Veterinary medicine: an illustrated history. St. Louis: Mosby; 1996. p. 556–61.

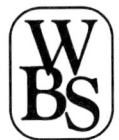
Vet Clin Food Anim 18 (2002) 197–205

THE VETERINARY
CLINICS
Food Animal
Practice

Index

Note: Page numbers of article titles are in **boldface** type.

A

Agricultural products, introduction of disease by way of, 184–185

Animal products, introduction of disease by way of, 184–185

Animals, other than cattle, import of, 119

Animate vectors, of enteric infectious agents, importance of, 21–22

Antibiotics, for treatment of intramammary infections, 116, 117–118

Antimicrobials, effectiveness of, 2
  resistance to, 2

Arthropod-borne diseases, biosecurity for, **99–114**
  biosecurity risk assessment for, 103–113
  exposure assessment, 103–104
  hazard identification, 103
  host ecology of, 101
  identification of mitigations lessening, 105–109, 111, 112–113
  of North America, 102–103
  pathogen ecology of, 101
  risk assessment for, 104–105, 109
  vector ecology of, 100–101

B

Babesiosis, eradication of, 99–100

Biocontainment, 178–179, 188
  biosecurity and, epidemiologic tools for, **155–173**
  creation of spreadsheet model of, 158
  definition of, 1
  domestic, bovine practitioner's role in, 192
  goal of, 155
  modeling aggregate testing strategies for, 167–172
  modeling diagnostic tests of, 157–160
  modeling probability of event in, 161
  modeling results of surveys of, 160–161
  models of, examples of, 158–160
  principles of, 155
  quantitative models of, 155–156

Changing Your Address?

Make sure your subscription changes too! When you notify us of your new address, you can help make our job easier by including an exact copy of your Clinics label number with your old address (see illustration below.) This number identifies you to our computer system and will speed the processing of your address change. Please be sure this label number accompanies your old address and your corrected address—you can send an old Clinics label with your number on it or just copy it exactly and send it to the address listed below.

We appreciate your help in our attempt to give you continuous coverage. Thank you.

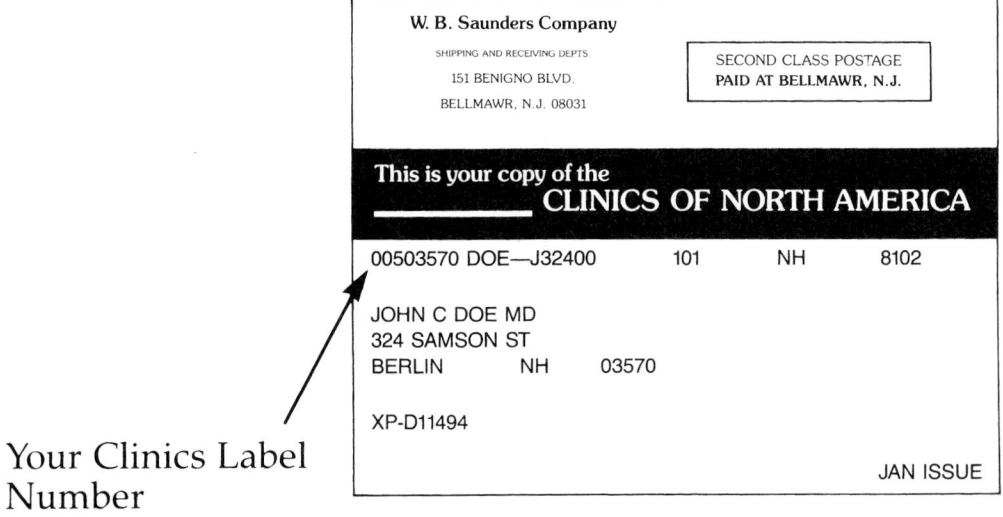

W. B. Saunders Company

SHIPPING AND RECEIVING DEPTS.
151 BENIGNO BLVD.
BELLMAWR, N.J. 08031

SECOND CLASS POSTAGE
PAID AT BELLMAWR, N.J.

This is your copy of the
_____ **CLINICS OF NORTH AMERICA**

00503570 DOE—J32400   101   NH   8102

JOHN C DOE MD
324 SAMSON ST
BERLIN   NH   03570

XP-D11494

JAN ISSUE

Your Clinics Label Number
Copy it exactly or send your label along with your address to:
W.B. Saunders Company, Customer Service
Orlando, FL 32887-4800
Call Toll Free 1-800-654-2452

Please allow four to six weeks for delivery of new subscriptions and for processing address changes.